D1356187

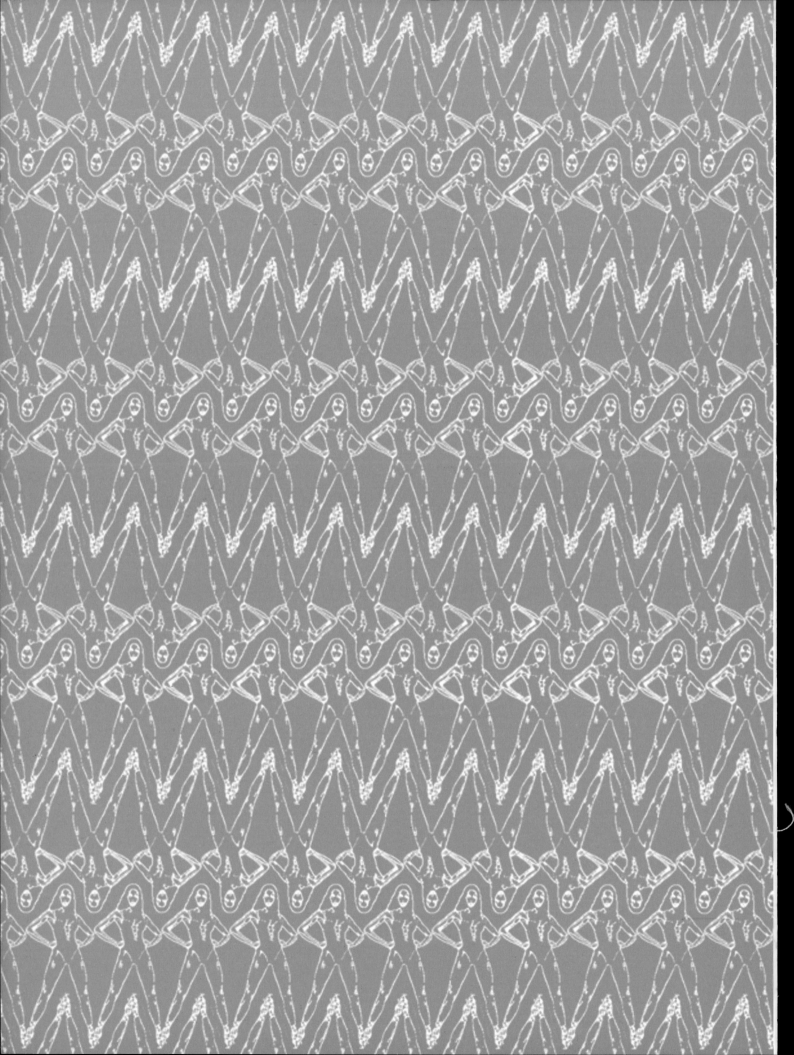

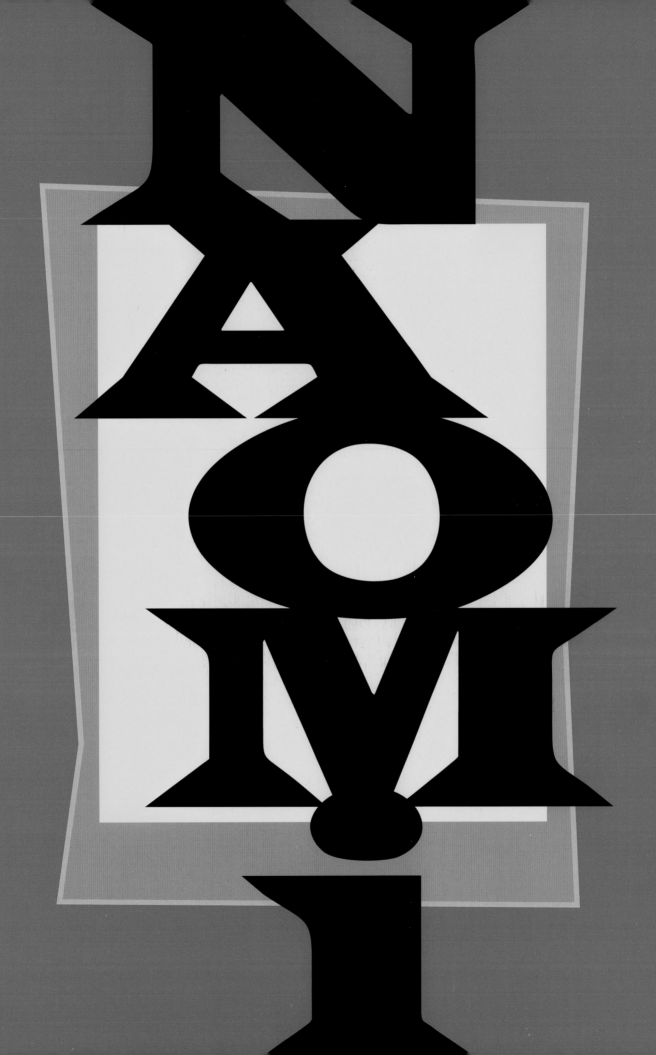

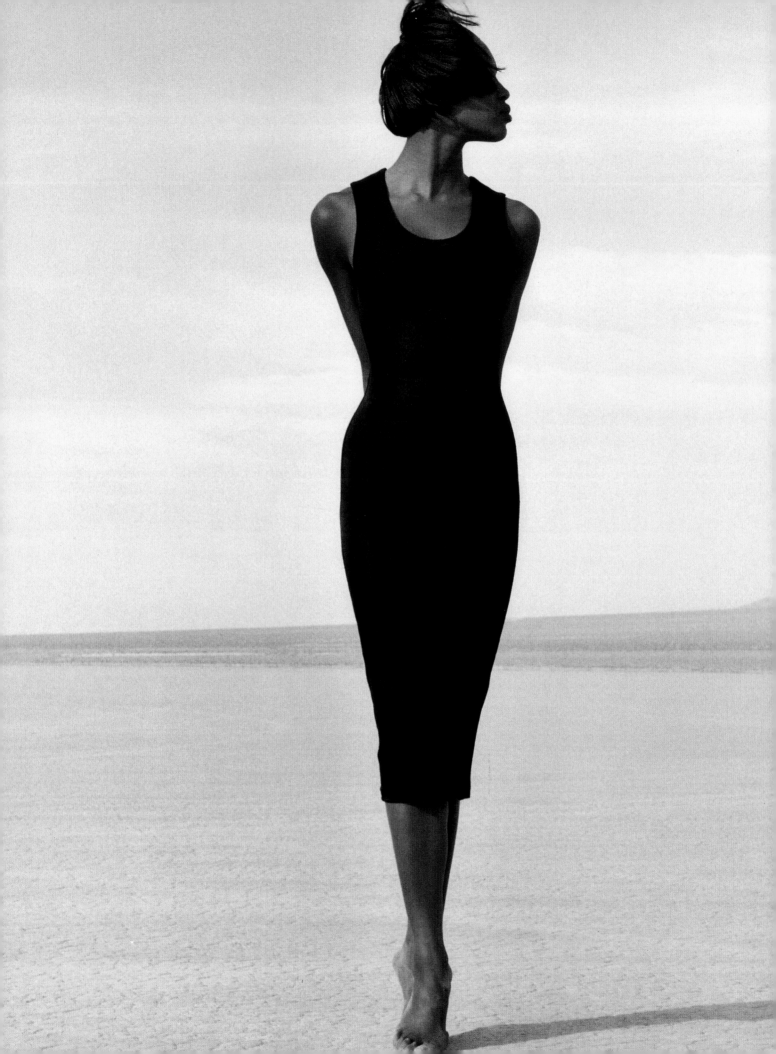

NAOMI Naomi Campbell

Herb Ritts
El Mirage, 1988
Vogue

HAMLYN

All of Naomi Campbell's proceeds from
the sale of this book will benefit the
Somali Red Crescent Society, part of the
International Federation of Red Cross
and Red Cross Societies.

First published in the United Kingdom in 1996 by Hamlyn,
an imprint of Reed Consumer Books Limited,
Michelin House, 81 Fulham Road,
London SW3 6RB
and Auckland, Melbourne, Singapore and Toronto

Copyright © 1996 London Kilt, Inc.
All Rights Reserved.

No part of this publication may be reproduced,
stored in a retrieval system, or transmitted in
any form or by any means, electronic, mechanical,
photocopying, recording, or otherwise, without
prior consent of the publishers.

A Catalogue record for this book is available from the
British Library
ISBN 0 600 59109 3

Design by Bruce Ramsay

Design assistance by Matthew Guemple,
Daniel Pfeffer, and John Giordani

Printed in Italy

Cover photograph
Michael Thompson
New York, 1994
Allure

Back cover photograph
Herbie Knott
Paris, 1993
Vivienne Westwood Show

Thierry Le Goùes
1992
Vogue Homme

Following spread
Steven Sebring
New York, 1996

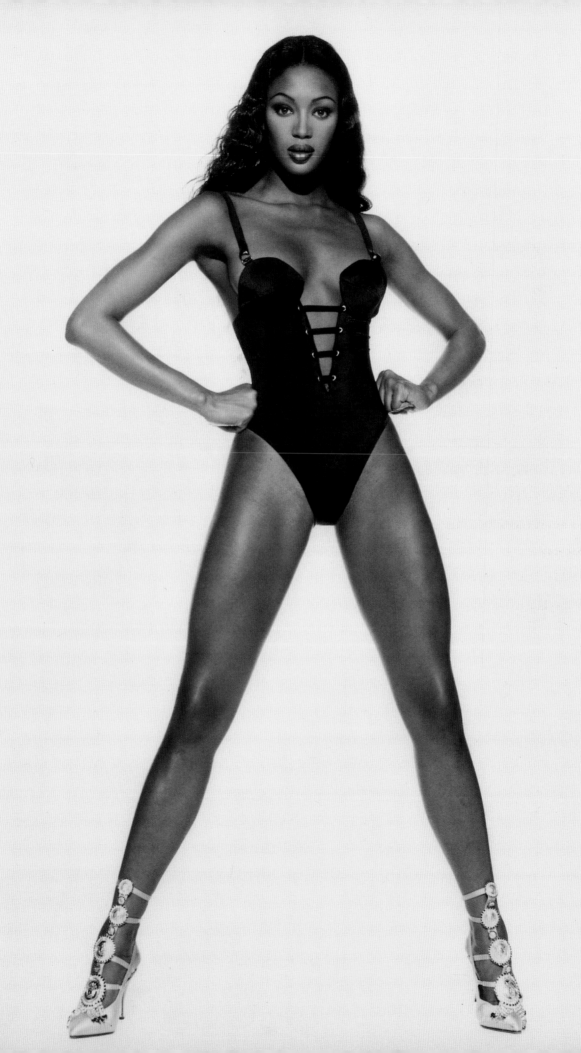

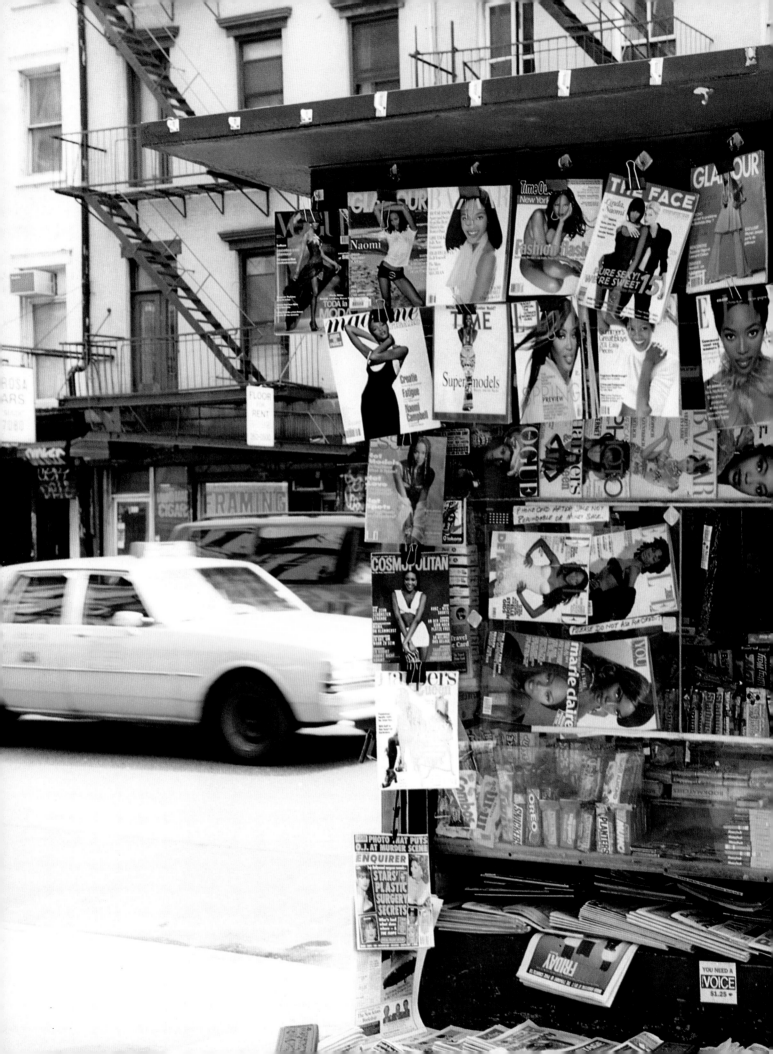

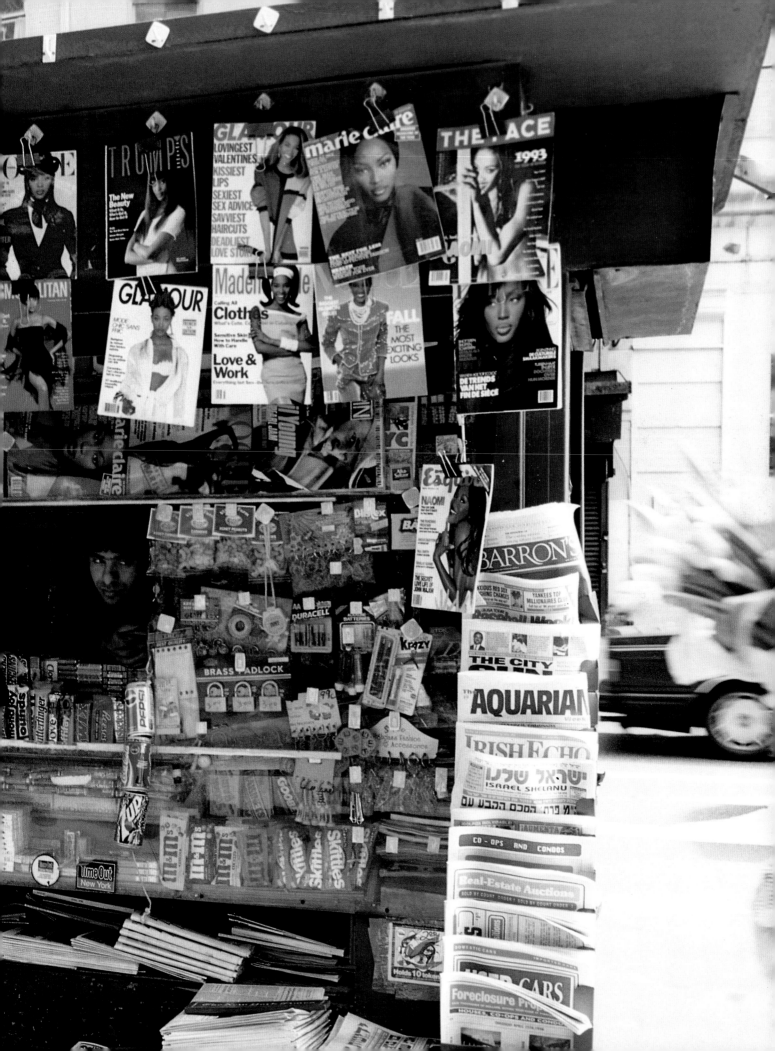

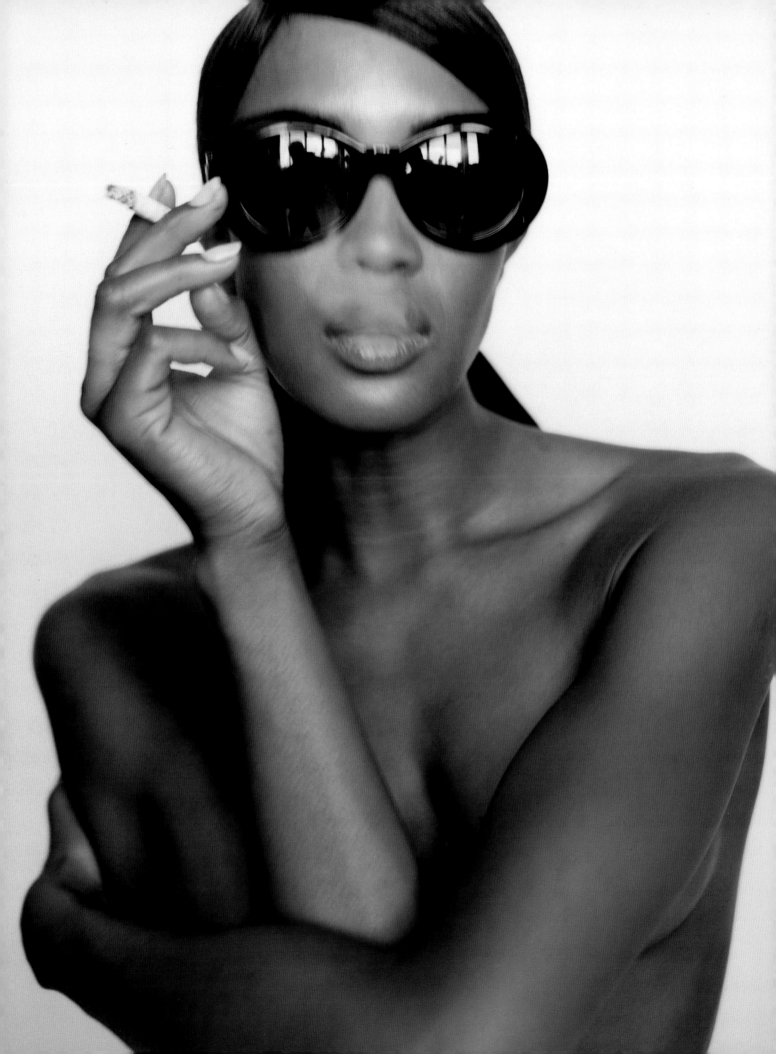

Contents

Mario Testino
Paris, 1995
Versace campaign

On February 13, 1996 I received a fax from Naomi requesting me to write a 500-word foreword to a photo book she was putting together... and the deadline was February 24, 1996!

Upon receipt I called her assistant to inform her that I would have to pass, due to the short deadline.

But I was not off the hook.

She immediately replied, "Take an extra week!"

On February 24, 1996, in the sanctuary of my Switzerland home–away from any fashion scene, gossip, or tabloid journalism–I started writing about Naomi.

I first met Naomi backstage at a Thierry Mugler show in the mid-80s. It was one of her first shows...and one of my last.

"Why do you hate me?" she asked.

"Why should I hate you, I don't even know who you are," I replied.

I knew right then that she had the makings of a diva! She was already making herself important. The trick was not lost on me. I instantly liked her.

Naomi is friendlier, funnier and sweeter than one would possibly imagine and upon meeting her one cannot resist her transparent girlishness.

She is a 5' 9½" sculpted African beauty who crashed the New York fashion scene in the early 80s, via London. She has a black dancer's body: muscled, but long and lean. On any given day she could have beautiful dark brown, hazel, green or blue eyes. On any given catwalk, she could have dark, short cropped, golden shoulder length, jet black, below the waist, or dead-straight hair. At any given moment, she totally reinvents herself.

I could almost suffocate her with sociological significances, from her "unapolegetic" West African features, her complete disregard for convention, her defiant appropriation of couture–spoils of war rarely won by a "sister"–to her equally sassy monopoly of some of the most desirable males around (my husband excepted, of course). She has simply galvanized her profession into unveiling more ethnicity, more cultural cross-over, and more willingness to move away from the white stereotype.

When I arrived on the fashion scene in the late 70s, I may have opened a number of doors, but this was due in large part to my fine, typically Somali features.

Naomi swept in at the start of a whole new era of awareness. The currency was hybridization. The vocabulary was splashed with Hip-Hop, Basquiat, Black dance, The Jacksons–Michael and Jessie and global anything! The afro-awareness in the U.S. was never so ripe for the pure, uncompromised looks of this new girl on the block. In reality Naomi didn't have to change a thing about herself. Things were changing around her and all she had to do was walk that walk...!

The fashion industry is engaged in the production of images, and at times its views have been colored by prejudice. Photography is a mirror in which we see ourselves reflected. Naomi gave a lot of young black women a supportive and beautiful reflection.

Her beauty self-evident, sex appeal unsurpassed, and her modeling success unmitigated...

All that is left to say is...you go girl!

FOREWORD BY IMAN

Paolo Roversi
Paris, 1994
Pigalle, unpublished

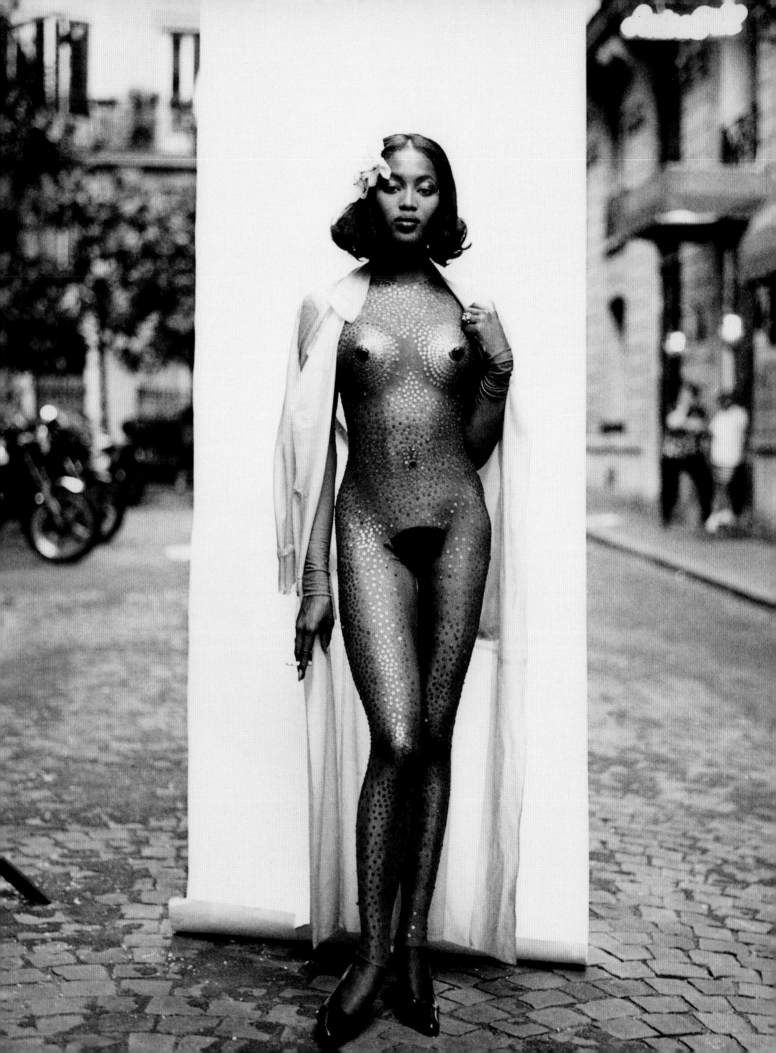

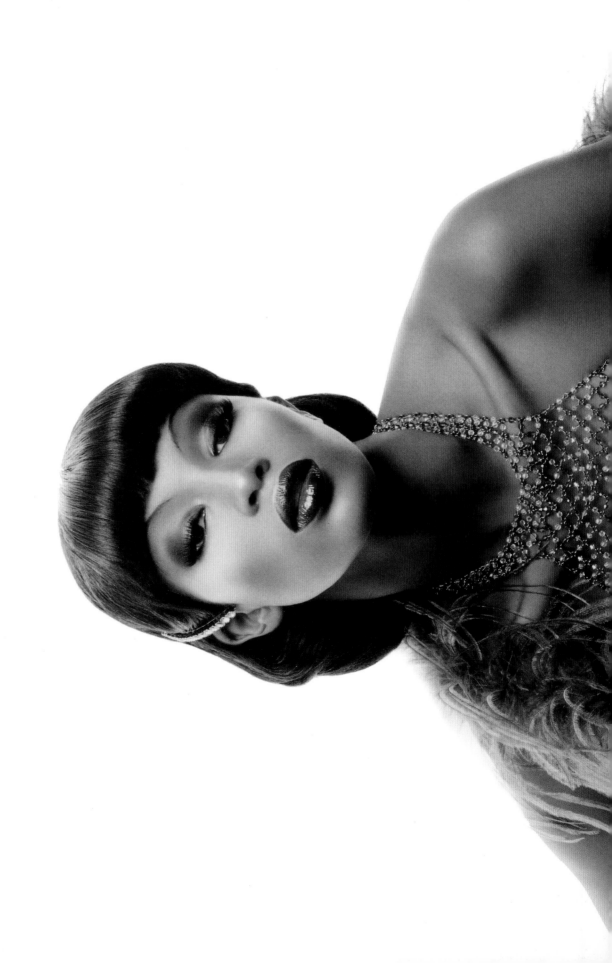

Matthew Rolston
New York, 1994
Spanish Vogue

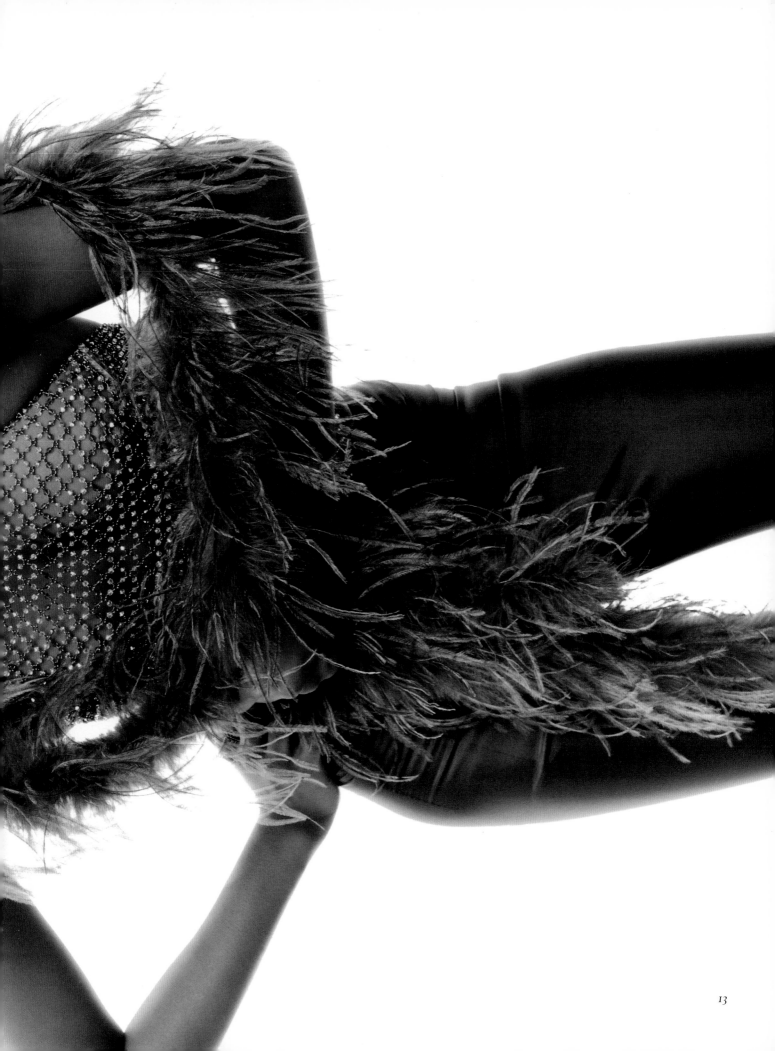

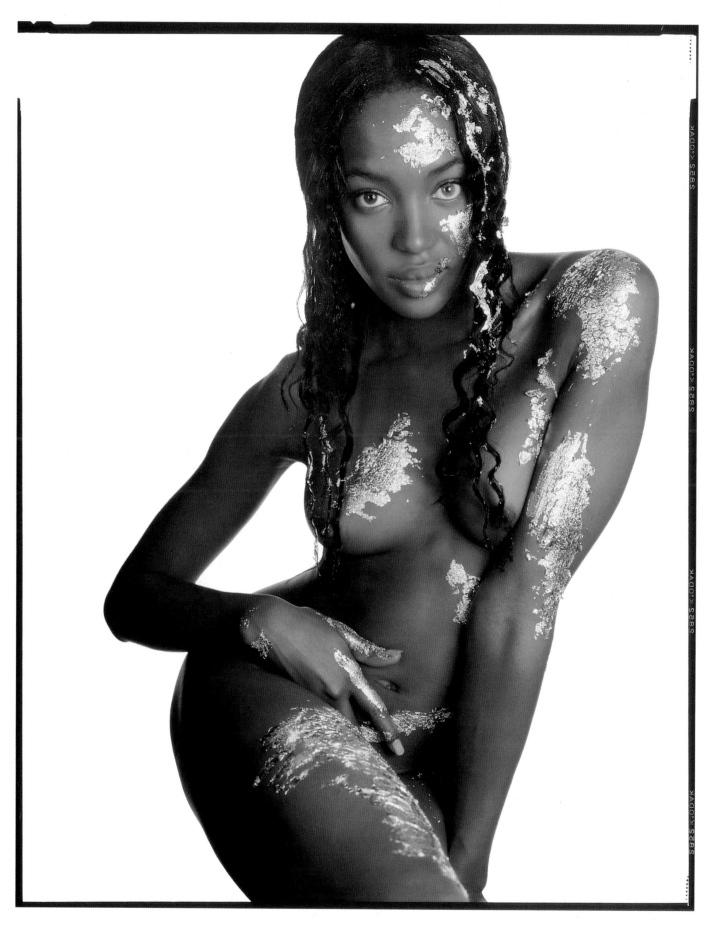

Richard Avedon
© 1995, Pirelli/Avedon
Pirelli

Naomi Campbell is like a beautiful pearl resting on top of a lush black velvet background.

There is an age-old saying that beauty is only skin deep. But in the case of Naomi Campbell, beauty begins down in the depths of the heart. I have been fortunate over the course of my life to have met many people who possess that innate trait, which embraces everyone who comes into contact with them, and Naomi is definitely one of those people. She exudes an electric energy and warmth when she walks into a room, lighting it up like the New York skyline on a clear summer night.

When I first met Naomi, I could tell right away that there was more to her than just a pretty face. It was obvious that her intellect matched her talents, and I knew that she was a rising star about to break loose. The discipline which she learned as a child while studying dance, singing, and acting, has molded Naomi into a magnificent presence. Possessing a purity and appreciation for every aspect of life, the uniqueness which is Naomi Campbell is that she doesn't really know how wonderfully talented she is.

Having captured the world's attention at the young age of sixteen, Naomi has let nothing stand in the way of achieving her goals. After gracing the covers of the world's most glamorous magazines, she first appeared on screen in Michael Jackson's *In the Closet* video. And I know she will conquer the big screen when she appears in the films *Miami Rhapsody*, *Girl 6*, and *Invasion of Privacy*. She has successfully parlayed her high-profile modeling career into leading roles in films, and a singing career—she appears on the "Heaven's Girl" track on my latest album, *Q's Jook Joint*—and now with the opening of Fashion Cafe, business. And I am sure that the success that she has had in everything that she has endeavored to do will continue, because she will work at it until it does.

When I think of Naomi, "supermodel" doesn't seem to be the appropriate title. The more apt title would be "superperson." She has taken her God-given talents and is successfully using them to continually grow, and I am looking forward to her maturing into a successful entrepreneur. She has the humility and grace to last a very long time in this business. And in this business, longevity is synonymous with success.

And, in case anyone mistakes Naomi for being monodynamic, her range should never be underestimated. She has the full capacity to go from "Pianissimo" to "Fortissimo." But most of all, she is like one of my cherished daughters and I treasure our friendship. So take a trip through this book about her charmed life. You'll like it a lot.

INTRODUCTION BY QUINCY JONES

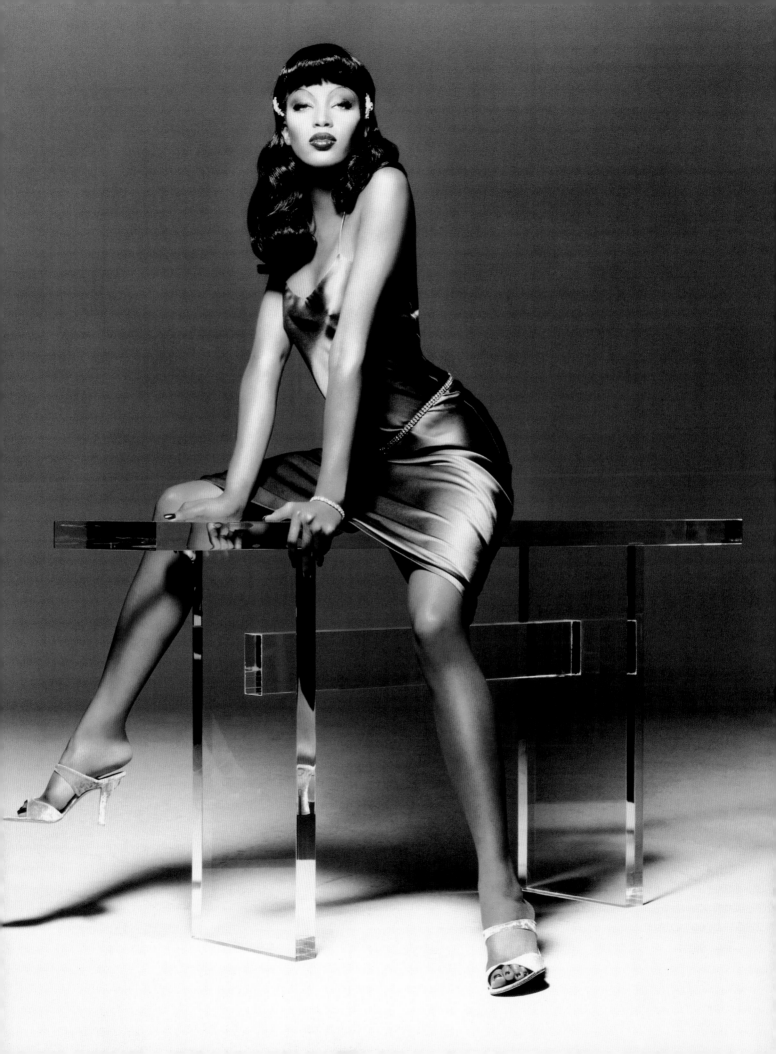

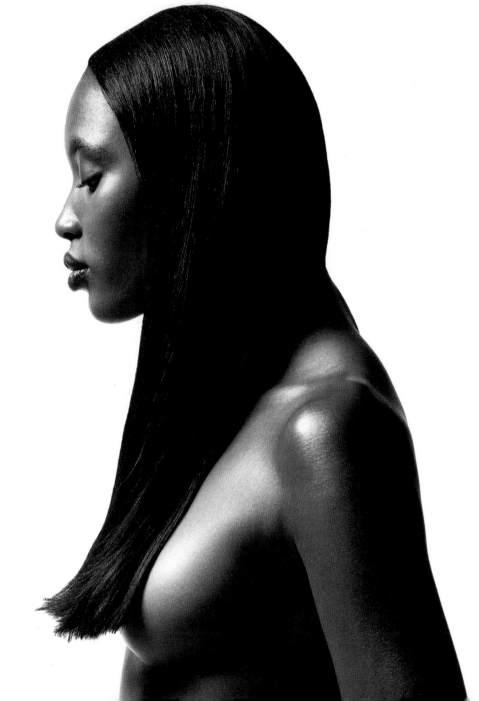

Thierry Le Gouès
1994
unpublished

Opposite
Matthew Rolston
New York, 1994
Spanish Vogue

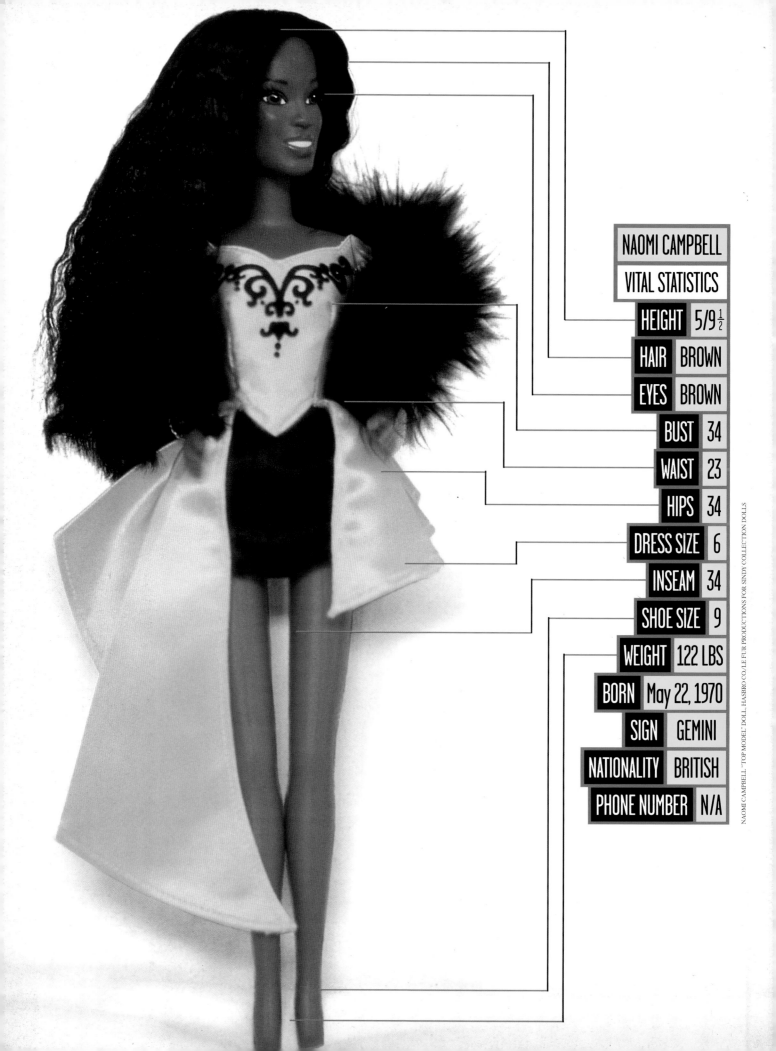

NAOMI CAMPBELL	
VITAL STATISTICS	
HEIGHT	5/9 ½
HAIR	BROWN
EYES	BROWN
BUST	34
WAIST	23
HIPS	34
DRESS SIZE	6
INSEAM	34
SHOE SIZE	9
WEIGHT	122 LBS
BORN	May 22, 1970
SIGN	GEMINI
NATIONALITY	BRITISH
PHONE NUMBER	N/A

NAOMI CAMPBELL "TOP MODEL" DOLL, HASBRO CO./LE FUR PRODUCTIONS FOR SINDY COLLECTION DOLLS

NAOMI ON NAOMI

An Interview

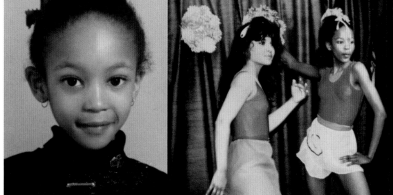

NAOMI, CAN YOU TELL ME SOMETHING ABOUT YOUR CHILDHOOD AND YOUR FAMILY?

I went to a school of theater arts from five to sixteen. I danced and studied theater every single day. Basically, my mother was a dancer, so I traveled a lot as a child—since I was three weeks old. I was brought up in Italy, then in Switzerland, and I had a pretty good childhood. I had a very tough mother, she's very supportive. She's young, but whatever I choose to do, she's there and she tries to help me.

I've got a big family. I mean, I only have one brother—he's named Pierre—but I have a huge extended family. My mother has nine, er, eight brothers and sisters. So I have tons of cousins and uncles.

You have no other brothers and sisters?

No. Just my brother—we have fifteen and a half years between us. He's only ten.

And where is he?

He's in London. He lives here and my mother lives here. Most of our family lives here, and the rest live in Jamaica. My family's originally Jamaican, but my grandfather's from Sheffield, England, and my grandmother is part Chinese on my real father's side. Her name, the family name, was Ming before Campbell. There's a big community of Jamaican-Chinese people.

How does it feel, knowing that many young African and African-American girls dream about you—many of them with the new Naomi doll at their bedside.

It's flattering to me to have young African or African-American women, any ethnic culture, look up to me or consider me a role model. The thing is, I don't want to be a role model just because I'm a model. I would like to be a role model for doing something that's worthy, for doing something for the community, for giving something back. So there are a number charities I'm involved in.

And the doll—I'm getting kind of used to the idea. From the profile it looks like me, from the front I'm not so sure.

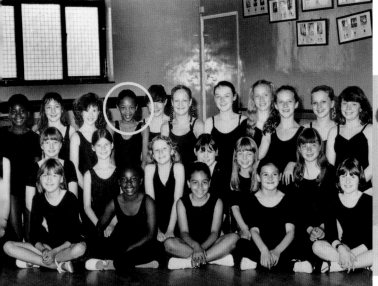

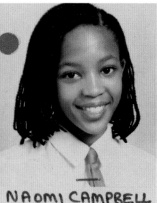

NAOMI CAMPBELL

• Clockwise from top: Naomi's school picture at age six; Naomi performing at the Barbara Speake Stage School, London, 1984; Naomi's school picture at age eight; Rehearsal class for the Royal Variety Performance at the Barbara Speake Stage School, London, 1979
• Opposite page, clockwise from top: Iman and Naomi at Thierry Mugler show, 1990; Naomi's birthday party at Laura Belle (l to r: Naomi, Steven Meisel, and Madonna), New York, 1991; Karen Mulder, Naomi, and Claudia Schiffer, holding their "Top Model" dolls, Paris, 1996; Tribute to Warner Bros. Studio (l to r: Christy Turlington, Quincy Jones, Naomi, and Yasmeen Ghauri), Los Angeles, 1991

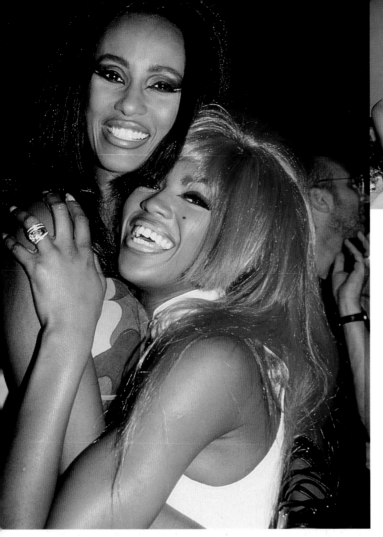

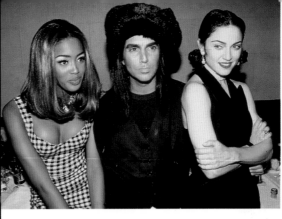

CLOCKWISE FROM TOP: ROXANNE LOWIT; BUTLER/BAUER/REX USA LTD; PATRICK DEMARCHELIER/SYGMA; GILLES BASSIGNAC/GAMMA LIAISON

Who did you look up to as a young girl?

For me, I think the one lady I've always admired before I became a model—and I've had the pleasure of meeting her—is Iman, who is Somali. She was very, very supportive of me and she was very helpful. I still admire her; I think she's a lady with great elegance and intelligence.

Is it difficult to be a model?

Sometimes the traveling is pretty hard. It's difficult and rewarding in many different ways. I've gotten into many different business deals and licensings, and I've met wonderful people. And I have many great opportunities just because I'm in this business. I know that if I wasn't, it wouldn't have come to me so easily.

Privacy is a very important thing to me, and that's very difficult in this business recently, because everyone's been very

focused on the fashion world all of a sudden, so everything we do is written down. It's like they've made us into these celebrities. And they focus so much on us and then pull it away sometimes. I think they're all very smart and they know that when we have the power we want to keep it. But power is something I don't think you should use just to promote yourself. You should also use it to speak out about things you believe in, because you know you have that public persona.

What does it take to be model?

I think you have to have a lot of ambition. In the right way, not the type where you want to tread on people. It's a different type of ambition: it's a goal, it's something you want to achieve, it's your long term future, it's what you want, it's discipline. You have to have a lot of drive.

There are good and bad moments. And you can't take things personally. I mean, if you go for a casting and you're not right for it, you just have to say, "Okay, I didn't get that job, there's something else for me. There's something else coming." It's difficult to learn. I learned actually when I was in London, when I was getting started, not to take things personally. Because you can, and it can be very upsetting. But I think that nowadays, the models that I know, we're all very business-minded. And we realize that we're in a very big business that makes a lot of money and that's how we think. We're a commodity to ourselves.

Now it's time for "alphabet confidential"—I give you a word beginning with a particular letter of the alphabet, and I'll ask you to give a quick response. First: "A" is for Africa. What does Africa mean to you?

Africa to me is a very mysterious place. I've only been to one part

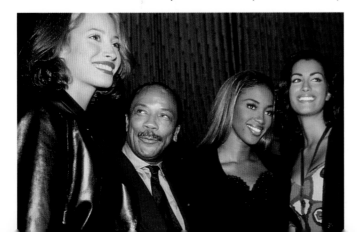

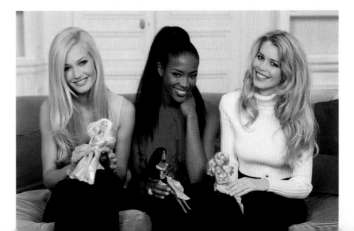

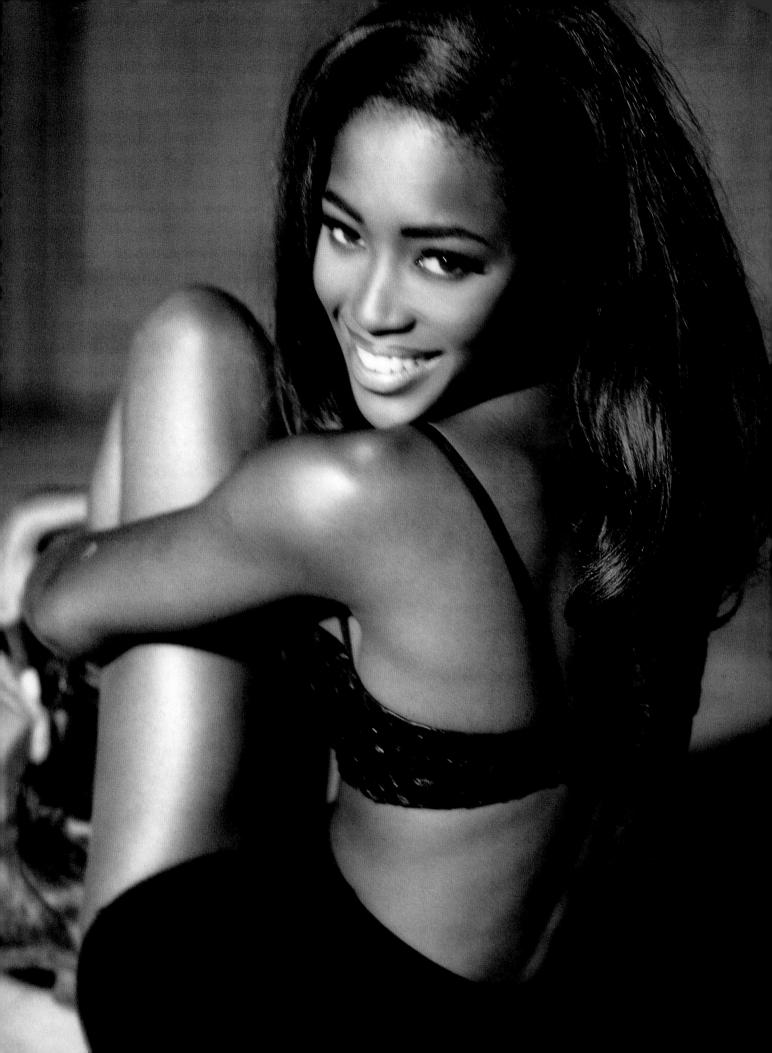

THERE IS ONLY ONE SUPERMODEL THAT STALKS THE CATWALKS OF PARIS, LONDON, NEW YORK, MILAN AND IT IS NAOMI CAMPBELL. SHE RULES. WHY? THE STYLE IS IN THE GENETIC FACTOR: THAT FIRM DERRIERE IS SO HIGH, SO STERN YOU COULD SIT A CHAMPAGNE FLUTE ON IT AND USE IT AS A COCKTAIL TABLE. NAOMI HAS ALL THE ADVANTAGES AND DISADVANTAGES OF A WOMAN OF COLOR. SHE HAS TO WORK FIVE TIMES AS HARD AS THE NEXT SOLDIERINE JUST TO STAY ON TOP. YET HER CAREER BLITZ IS UNIQUE: MUSIC, A GHOST-WRITTEN NOVEL, MOVIES, CAMEO VIDEO APPEARANCES, AND ALL THE GILDED STUFF THAT GOES WITH FAME. UNDERNEATH THAT VENEER OF GLAMOUR AND BLACK CHIC IS STILL A LITTLE GIRL WITH HER STUFFED TEDDY BEAR IN HER HAND, LOOKING FOR A REASSURING HAND TO PULL THE COVERS UP TO HER CHIN ON A FROSTY EVENING.

—ANDRE LEON TALLEY

Mark Liddell
George Michael's *Freedom 90*, 1990 video

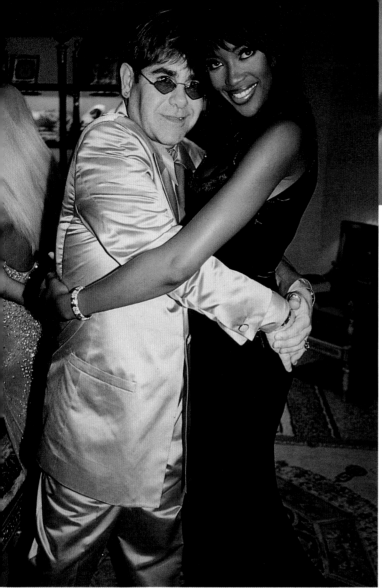

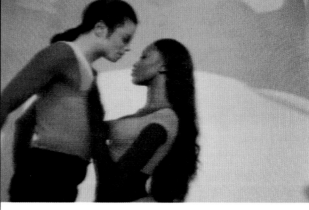

My favorite food is Jamaican food. It was what I was brought up on. And I find it to be very healthy at the same time. It makes me feel like I'm at home.

What type of food is there in Jamaica?

Chicken, plantains, mangos, all sorts of things.

Sounds a lot like African food.

Yes. One of my best friends from school is from Nigeria, and she's very, very smart. She's now going through her masters exam. Her name is Alison, and I remember having those things for dinner at her house. She's got a little baby, now. All my old school friends seem to have children now.

Why don't you have any children?

I don't want a child right now. I have too much to do, and when I do have children, I want to give them my utmost attention. I just want to make sure that security and everything is set up before I have a family.

"E" is for Elite. What does this word represent for you?

I'm with Elite in London and Paris. For me, they represent a good agency that understands what I want, what I want in my career. They work for me very well, and we work together for what we want to achieve.

"F" is for France. Do you have particular memories or souvenirs from France?

No but I'm getting one. I'm getting a medal from the Minister of Culture of France. I'll always remember that France was the first country to give me my *Vogue* cover.

"G" is for God. Are you religious. Do you believe in God?

I believe in God, but I'm religious for myself. I mean, I'm not a church-going person. I don't go every Sunday, but I pray at

of Africa, that's South Africa. It was very important for me to go there. I went there and met Mr. Mandela. He's the only person I've ever really wanted to meet.

"B" is for Beauty. What does beauty mean to you?

It can be within anybody. It's not just face value. It's something that you have inside that comes out.

"C" is for Celebrity. Is the celebrity life difficult to manage?

It's okay. It's just difficult when people invade your privacy. I just think you should never be famous just for the sake of being famous. You should be famous for doing something that's well-remembered.

"D" is for Delicious. What is your favorite food?

• Clockwise from top: Naomi with Elton John at Gianni Versace party, Daphnes, London, 1995; Naomi in Michael Jackson's *In the Closet* video, 1992; Elle Macpherson, Claudia Schiffer, and Naomi in the kitchen of the Fashion Cafe, New York, 1995 • Opposite page, clockwise from top: Naomi and Kate Moss in an elevator, New York, 1994; Spike Lee and Naomi on the set of *Girl 6*, 1996; Naomi, Isaac Mizrahi, and Linda Evangelista during the making of *Unzipped*, New York, 1995; Front and back covers of *Swan*, Naomi's other book, 1994

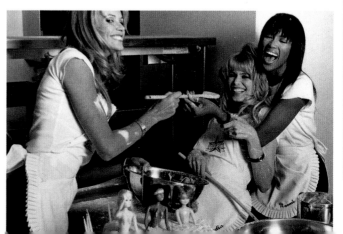

CLOCKWISE FROM TOP: RICHARD YOUNG/REX USA LTD; EVAN AGOSTINI/GAMMA LIAISON; THIERRY LE GOUÉS

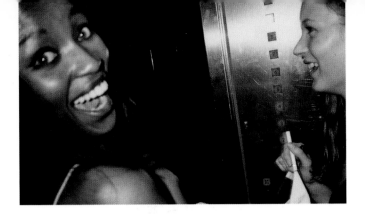

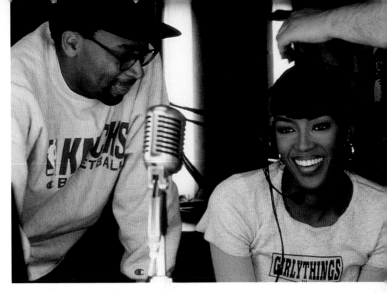

certain times, when I need strength from somewhere.

"H" is for Harmony. Do you find harmony in what you do? I also mean musically—you've recently put out an album.

I find harmony in music in general. I love to have music around me, I love to listen to music. I think it calms my temperament. It sets a certain tone. And my own music—I'm not totally satisfied with my music.

Why aren't you satisfied with your music?

Because it's my first album, and you learn, and it's an experience. And now that I've gone through the experience of doing my first album, there are a few things I'd like to change when I do a second one.

A second one?

I have no idea when I'll have time to do a second album, but I have to find time, because I'm still signed to Sony.

You also worked on a video for Michael Jackson. What did you think?

I like Michael Jackson. I had a great experience doing the video, and I had lots and lots of fun. He's very professional; he's a perfectionist in what he does and how he sees ideas in his mind visually. And I was very happy to work with him.

"I" is for Introverted. Are you a shy person?

Sometimes. Sometimes I can be an extrovert, sometimes I can be an introvert. It depends.

When?

Oh, I don't know. When I go to new places. You're not quite sure what to expect. You get nervous. Sometimes I go to a new restaurant, and it takes me fifteen minutes to get through the door. It depends. It doesn't really matter who I'm meeting.

"J" is for Jealousy. Do you ever get jealous?

I get jealous mostly when it has something to do with my personal life. Like with my boyfriend.

Can you give me the name of your boyfriend?

No.

"K" is for Kilo. How do you watch your weight? Is it difficult?

I don't watch my weight. I don't own a scale. I don't even look at one. I mean, I think that genetically, my family is lucky. We just don't really gain weight.

Do you eat a lot?

I eat all the time. It's a myth about models. All the models eat.

"L" is for Luxury. Do you like to live in luxury?

Once you get used to being treated in a certain way, you want to be treated like that all the time. But yes, doing what I do has enabled me to live a nice life.

"M" is for Mother. Do you want to have children eventually?

I'd like to have two children. I'd like to adopt one. I think I'll be a

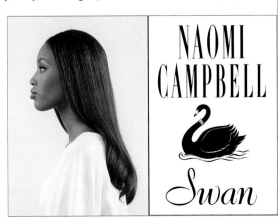

NAOMI
CAMPBELL

Swan

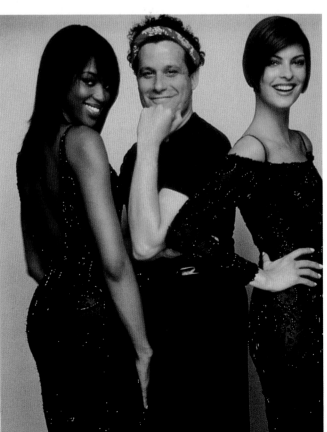

CLOCKWISE FROM TOP: CHRISTY TURLINGTON; DAVID LEE. ©FOX SEARCHLIGHT; PHOTOFEST; HUGGY RAGNARSSON

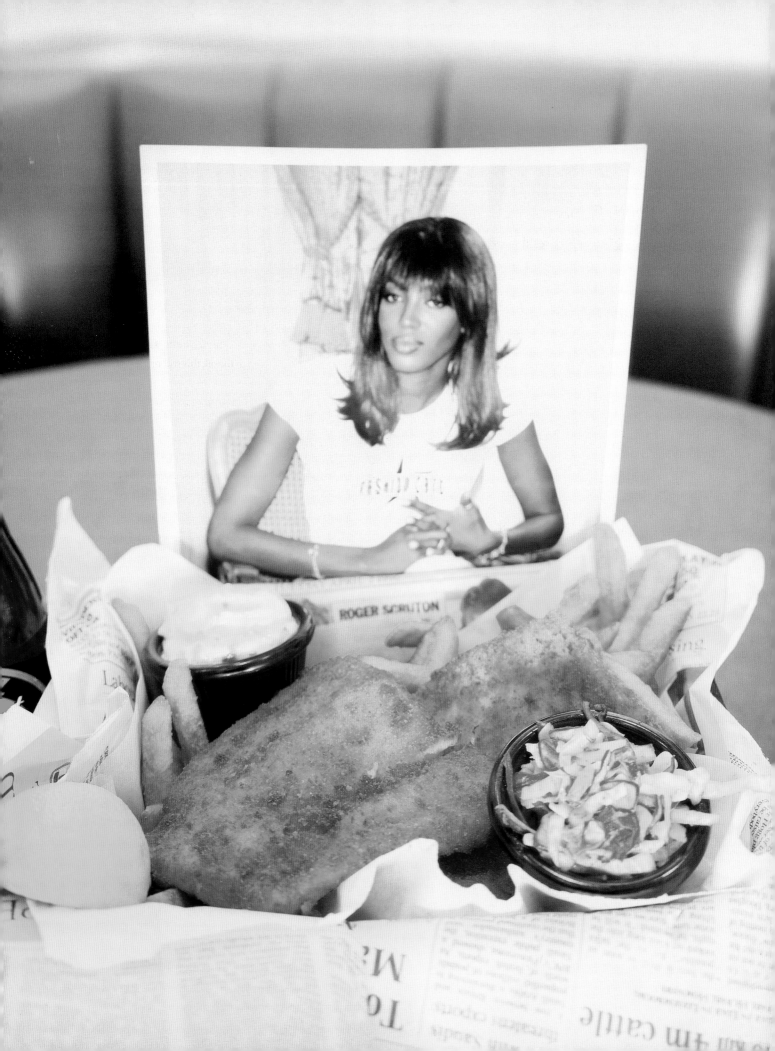

Fashion Cafe's Famous

Naomi's Fish & Chips

ingredients: *serves 4*

2 lbs. cod fish or plaice (where available)

juice of 1 large lemon

1 cup water

4 egg whites

2 cups bread crumbs

1 cup wheatgerm without honey (optional)

3 tsp garlic powder

3 scallions, diced fine

1 cup flour

vegetable oil (quantity varies depending on cooking method)

1.5 lbs medium russet potatoes or fries

pickled onions

tartar sauce

procedure:

1) Wash fish in lemon and water mixture.

2) Cut fish into 4 oz. pieces.

3) In a mixing bowl, beat egg whites until fluffy.

4) Mix bread crumbs, wheatgerm, garlic powder, and scallions in a bowl.

5) Lightly cover fish with flour (this ensures egg whites will stick to fish).

6) Coat each filet with egg whites and then dredge in bread crumb mixture.

7) Let fish sit for a couple of minutes in refrigerator.

cooking method I:

1) In a deep sauce pot, heat 1.5 quarts of oil to 350°.

2) Place fish carefully in hot oil. The fish should be completely covered. (Tip: If you have a strainer that fits inside the sauce pot, place the fish first inside it and then in the oil; this will make removal easier.)

3) Cook for 3-4 minutes.

4) Remove fish from oil and drain. Pat dry with a paper towel.

cooking method II:

1) In a sauté pan, heat 3 tbls. of vegetable oil.

2) Carefully place fish in pan.

3) Cook 2 minutes on each side, being careful while turning over.

4) Remove fish from pan and drain on a towel.

cooking potatoes:

1) Peel potatoes and slice into large pieces.

2) Heat oil to 350°.

3) Cook until golden brown.

4) Remove and drain.

helpful hints:

1) Use dry russet potatoes. New potatoes have too much water.

2) Par boil the potatoes before frying. Let drain and stand for one hour before cooking. This will help to achieve even cooking.

presentation:

Serve with pickled onions and tartar sauce in a grease-proof basket lined with English newspaper.

Adam Weiss
New York, 1996
Fashion Cafe

Naomi requires 100% attention and deserves it.
I look after her and try to keep up with her supersonic energy.
She has no boundaries.
She is intuitive and generous to a fault.
She has brains, beauty, style, and a body of pure perfection.
Her temper is like Tabasco.
She loves to love and be loved.

—Carole White

"Since I was three years old, I've been dancing. Now that I'm into modeling, I just can't let it go. Now I'm dancing and singing too."

—Naomi, from *Arthur Elgort's Models Manual*

Timothy White
New York, 1995
unpublished

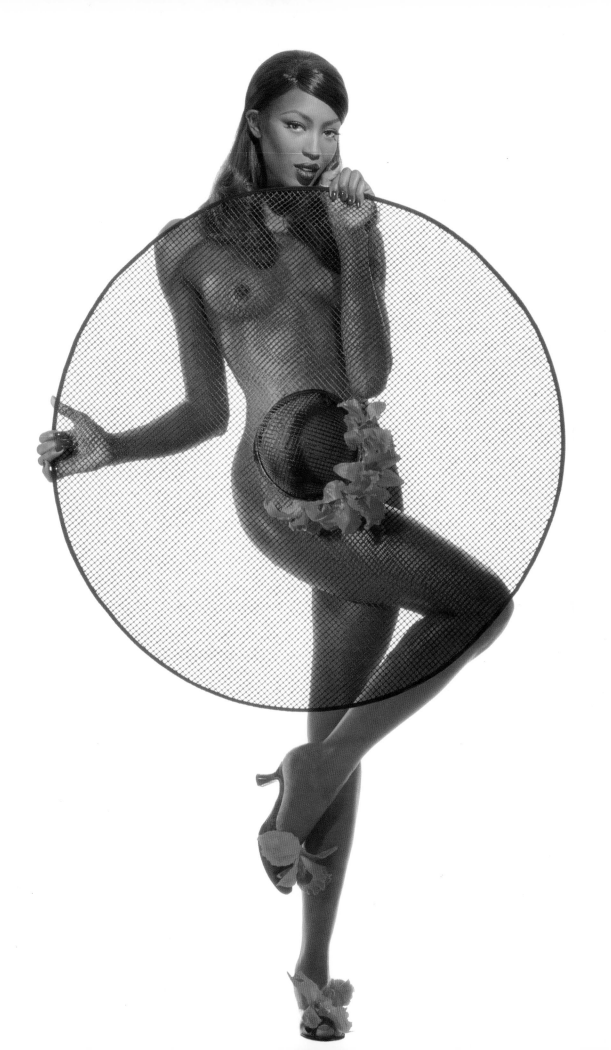

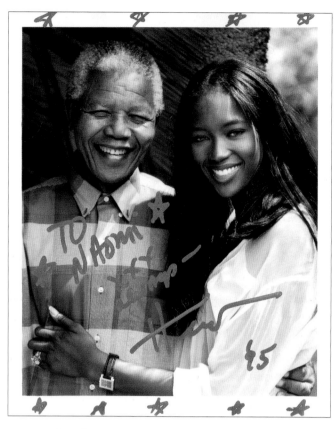

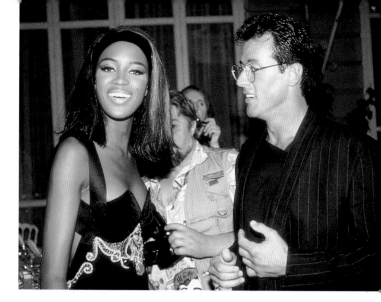

very good mother.

"N" is for Nerves. Are you a nervous person?

When I do shows. Just before I go onto the runway, I'm always very nervous.

"O" is for Organization. Are you very organized?

I'm a very organized person. Anyone who has to work with me can have a very hard time, because I want things done right away and I want things to be left where I put them.

"P" is for Poverty. Are you sensitive to the misery and poverty

around the world? How does it affect you?

Yes I am. I went to Poland once, and I went to a children's hospital, which was really devastating. Very sad. It makes you think you're very lucky, and you have to give back some of what you have.

"Q" is for Question. What are the most frequently asked questions you encounter?

What's it like to be model?

"R" is for Racism.

Racism for me is a challenge. And whenever someone says to me that something's not possible, I make it possible. It's a challenge, and a lot of things still have to change.

"S" is for Sex. You are a supreme sex symbol. How does this affect your personal life?

I think it's a pressure, because I'm not like that all the time. I think it's a fantasy that we make people believe. But in my regular life, I'm not like that. I just want to be me.

"T" is for Teenager. How do you see teenagers today? What do you think of child models?

I think child models are a little scary. It depends on if their family is supportive and involved. But I think you shouldn't start too young, that school should come first.

"U" is for Unity. Do you believe in the unity of the peoples of the world.

I do believe in unity, yes. I think that what's going on in Bosnia, Ethiopia, and Rwanda shows that people all over the world are trying to help solve these terrible problems that are right in

HITS OF THE WORLD

©1996, Billboard/BPI Communications

JAPAN (Dempa Publications Inc.) 06/10/96		
THIS WEEK	**LAST WEEK**	**SINGLES**
1	1	LA-LA-LA LOVE SONG TOSHINOBU KUBOTA WITH NAOMI CAMPBELL SONY
2	2	AINO KOTODAMA SPIRITUAL MESSAGE SOUTHERN ALL STARS VICTOR
3	3	REAL THING SHAKES B'Z ROOMS
4	NEW	BEAT YOUR HEART V 6 AVEX TRAX
5	4	ANATANI AITAKUTE SEIKO MATSUDA MERCURY MUSIC
6	5	ALICE MY LITTLE LOVER TOY'S FACTORY
7	7	CHERRY SPITZ POLYDOR
8	8	IIWAKE SYARANQ BMG VICTOR
9	6	KOKORO'O HIRAITE ZARD B-GRAM

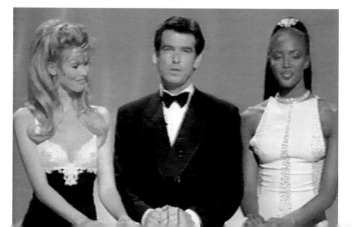

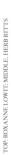TOP: ROXANNE LOWIT; MIDDLE: HERB RITTS

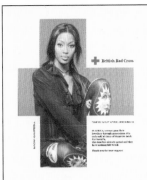

BRITISH RED CROSS
"Pot of Gold" Appeal for Somalia

IN AFRICA, women pass their jewellery through generations. It is only sold at times of desperate need. For Somalis, this time has already passed and they have nothing left to sell.

Thank you for your support.

• Clockwise from top: British Red Cross charity work in Somalia, advertising campaign, 1993; "Milk, What a surprise!" advertisement, 1995 • Opposite, clockwise from top: Naomi and Sylvester Stallone at Gianni Versace party, Hôtel Ritz, Paris, 1990; Costume Awards presentation at the 68th Annual Academy Awards (l to r: Claudia Schiffer, Pierce Brosnan, and Naomi), Los Angeles, 1996; Naomi with Nelson Mandela, South Africa, 1994

front of our faces.

"V" is for Vanishing. Do you see public respect for models vanishing today?

I think models are getting more respect now for the many different things they're involved in. As I've said, it's a business, it's on the rise every day. I think that we models are realizing what a growing business this is, so we're branching out. I have a restaurant with three other models, and I hope we'll branch out all over the world.

You're referring to Fashion Cafe. When did you open it?

The first one has opened in New York. The second is in New Orleans, the third in London, the fourth one in Barcelona, one in Paris, one in Jakarta.

Wow! How many in all?

Well, we're going to be opening seven this year. My partners are Elle Macpherson, Christy Turlington, and Claudia Schiffer.

"W" is for Wardrobe. What do you have in your wardrobe?

Do you have a Naomi "look"?

No I don't think I have a Naomi look, because I change my look all the time. The only thing you could say is my "look" is the brown pencil on my lips.

"X" is for X-Rated. Do you consider some of the work you do rather daring—such as the photograph in Madonna's book?

Doing the Madonna book was a great thing for her—letting people know her sexual fantasies. I know that people put sex under the carpet as a taboo subject, so I'm not ashamed that I did it. I know my family was a little upset, but that's okay. It's something I wanted to do.

"Y" is for You. What are your impressions of "you"? Have you achieved what you want to be?

I have achieved fifty percent of what I want to be. There's another fifty percent I'm still working towards achieving.

"Z" is for Zodiac. What's your sign?

I'm a Gemini.

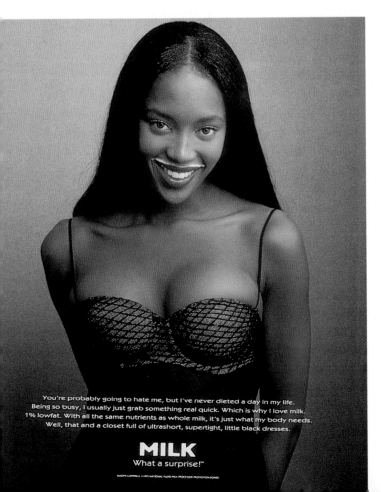

You're probably going to hate me, but I've never dieted a day in my life. Being so busy, I usually just grab something real quick. Which is why I love milk. 1% lowfat. With all the same nutrients as whole milk, it's just what my body needs. Well, that and a closet full of ultrashort, supertight, little black dresses.

MILK
What a surprise!"

NAOMI REPRESENTS AN ERA.
—BETHANN HARDISON

CLOCKWISE FROM TOP: HUGGY RAGNARSSON; ANNIE LEIBOVITZ FOR THE NATIONAL FLUID MILK PROCESSOR PROMOTION BOARD

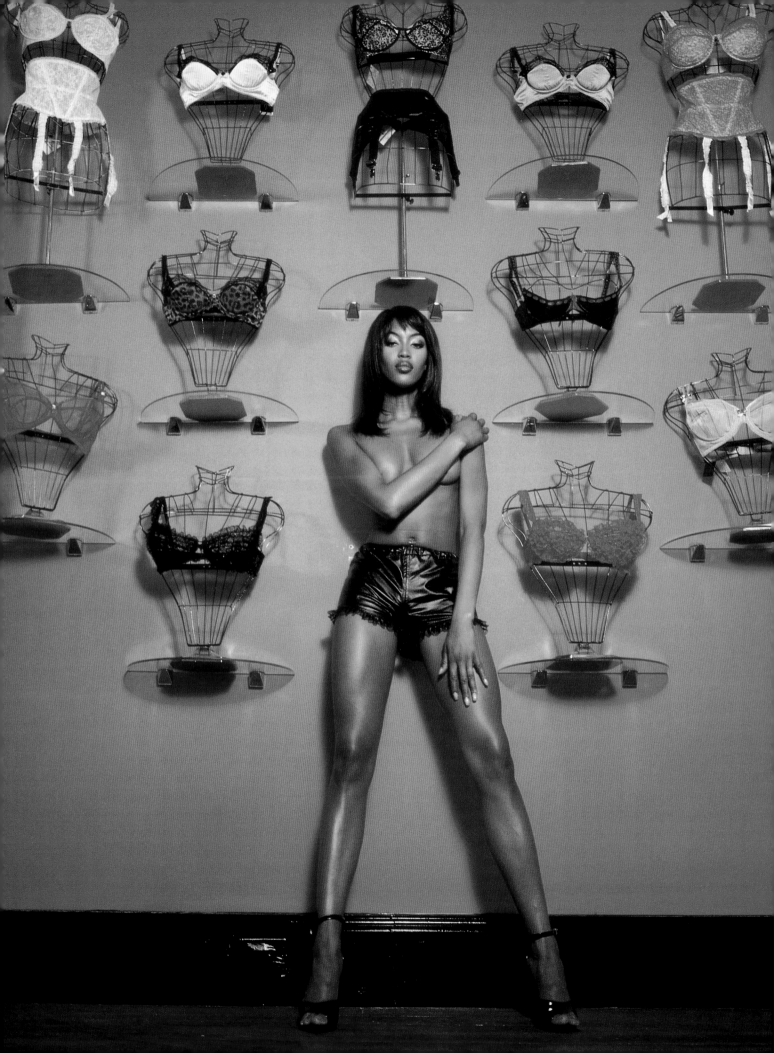

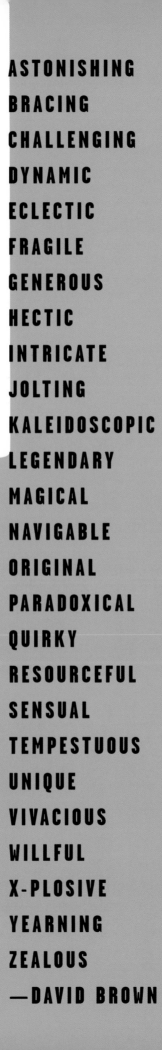

ASTONISHING
BRACING
CHALLENGING
DYNAMIC
ECLECTIC
FRAGILE
GENEROUS
HECTIC
INTRICATE
JOLTING
KALEIDOSCOPIC
LEGENDARY
MAGICAL
NAVIGABLE
ORIGINAL
PARADOXICAL
QUIRKY
RESOURCEFUL
SENSUAL
TEMPESTUOUS
UNIQUE
VIVACIOUS
WILLFUL
X-PLOSIVE
YEARNING
ZEALOUS
—DAVID BROWN

Huggy Ragnarsson
London, 1995
Agent Provocateur

David Letterman: Here now is Naomi Campbell at her best being a super-

model. Watch closely. You know what's frightening about that.

It looks like you could have broken both your ankles. **Naomi Campbell:**

I could have broken both my ankles.

DL: That was a nasty, nasty fall. **NC:** A terrible fall.

DL: But the other thing. Nobody moved to help you. **NC:** No one moved. No one moved a muscle in their faces. They were just nervous until I started laughing. And then they started laughing too. It didn't turn out that badly— I made an insurance commercial out of that.

CBS's *Late Show with David Letterman*, March 27, 1996

Herbie Knott
Naomi stumbles at the
Vivienne Westwood Show,
Paris, 1993

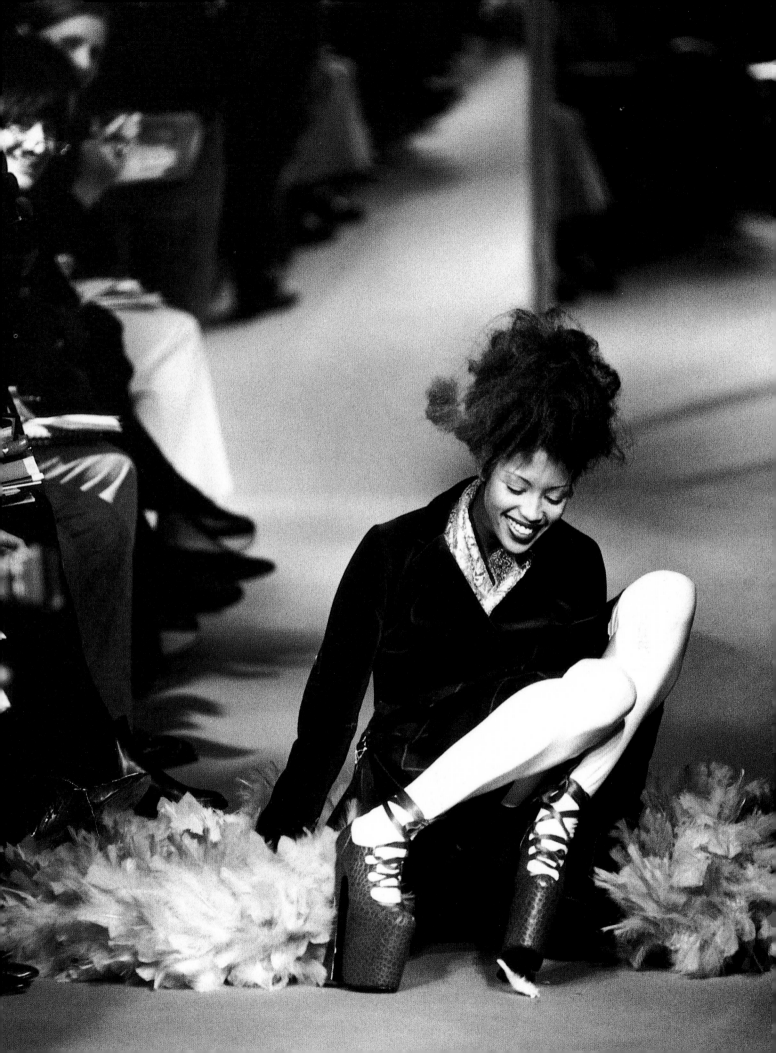

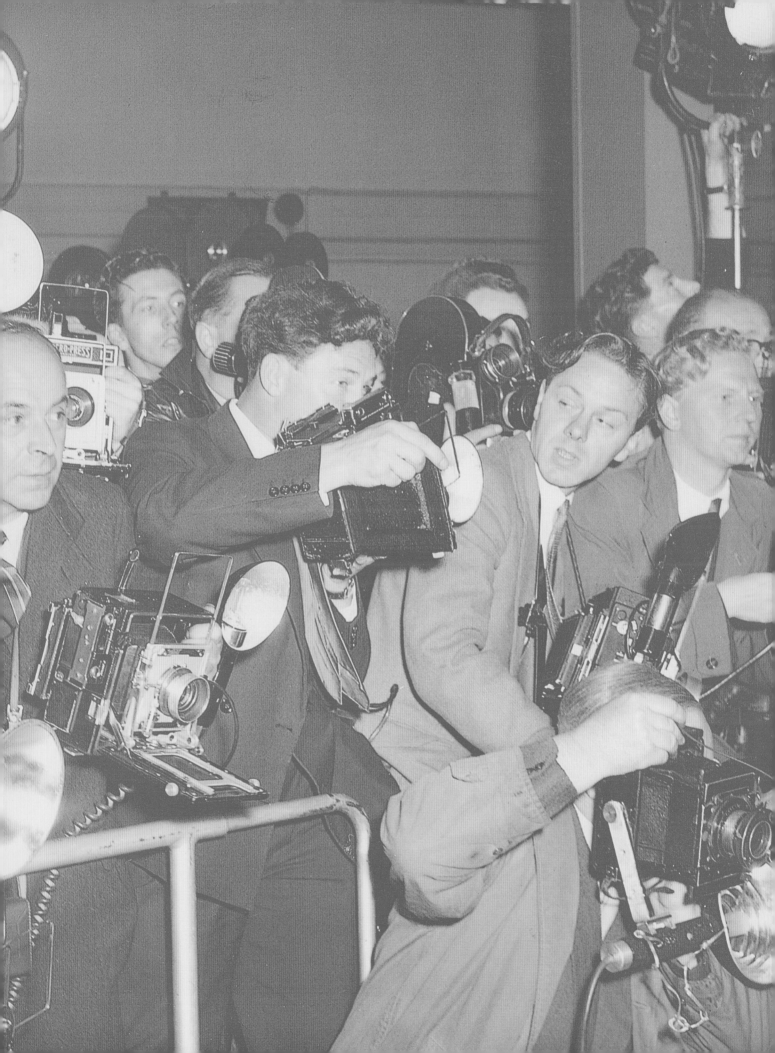

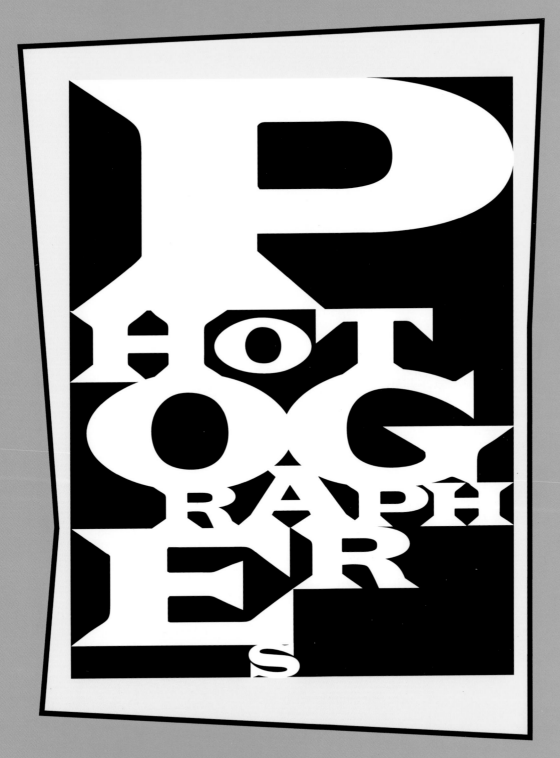

"When you're in front of the camera, you always have to

remember that you're modeling clothes. So I have to look good

in the outfit that I'm wearing. It's a collaboration between the photographer

and the hair and makeup people. I'm the end result of their work.

It's much better when you feel something from the photographer—

otherwise the picture comes out and I look lost."

–Naomi, from *Arthur Elgort's Models Manual*

Sante D'Orazio
1992
Italian Vogue

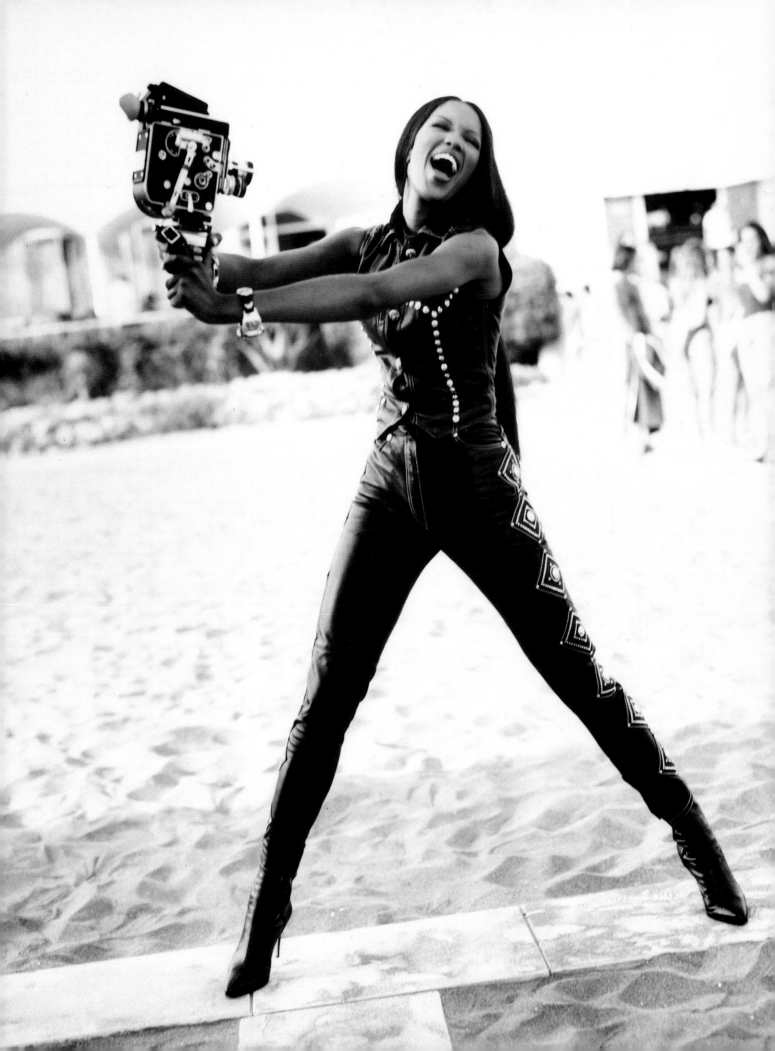

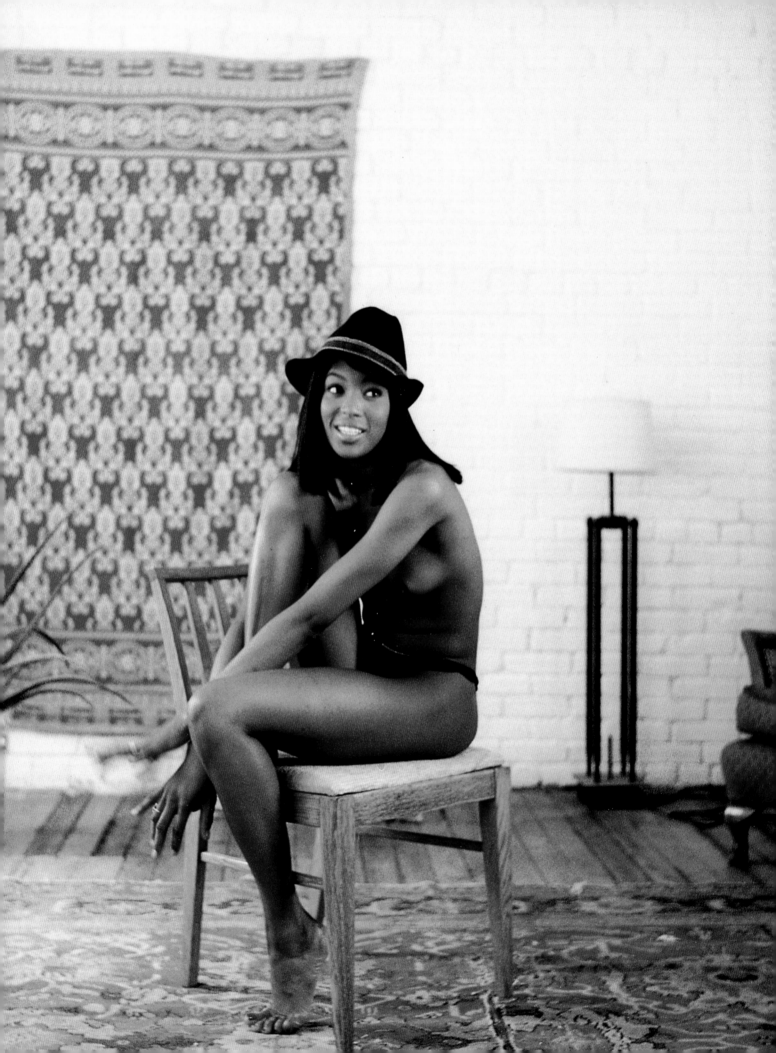

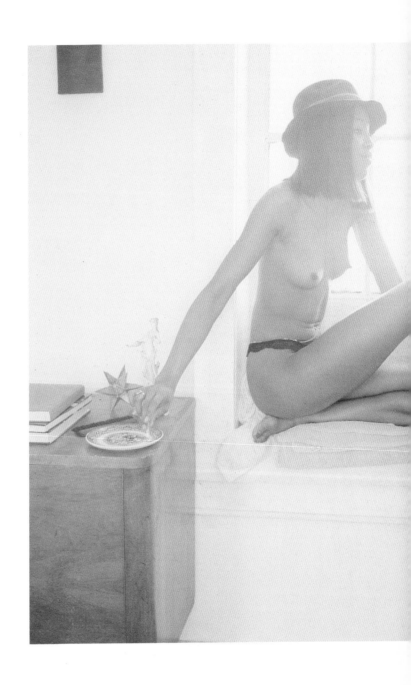

Jack Pierson
New York, 1994
unpublished

I ADORE NAOMI.
I ADORE NAOMI.
I ADORE NAOMI.
I ADORE NAOMI.
I ADORE NAOMI.
I ADORE NAOMI.

—Steven Meisel

When we say no to a photographer, or when a person
throws a mic in your face and you say no, you're
a bitch. You can't win. They're going to call you a bitch
either way. If I'm a bitch, I'm a hard-working bitch.
—Naomi, from *The Face*, 1994

Steven Meisel
1987
Italian Elle

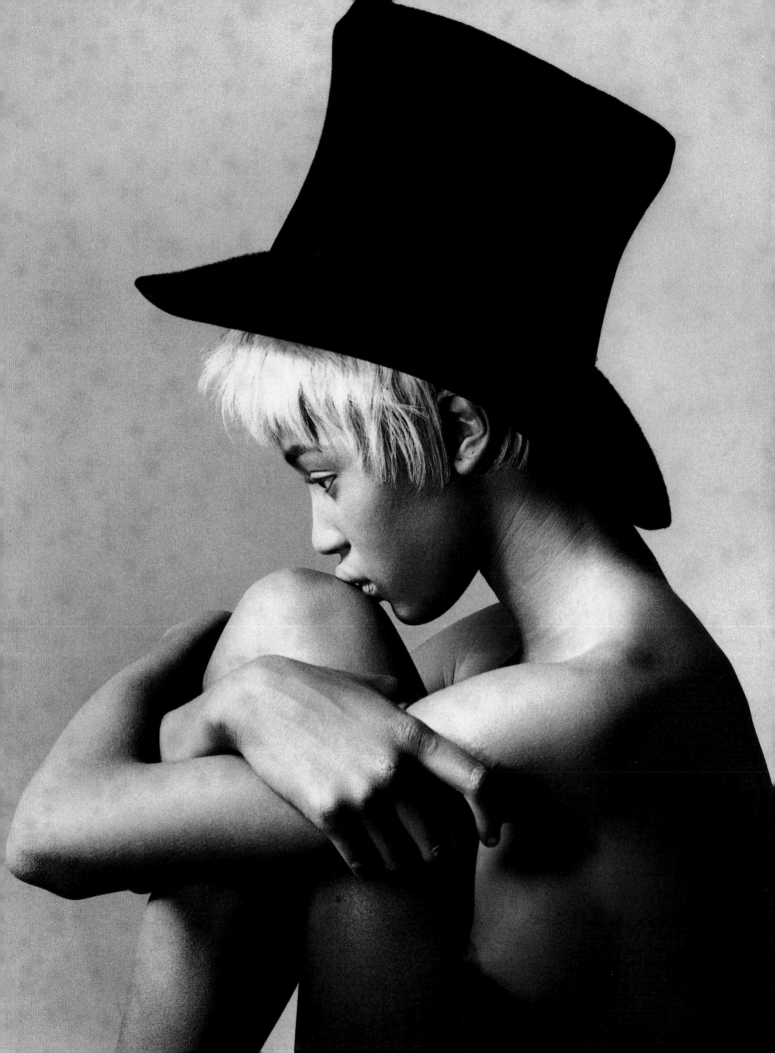

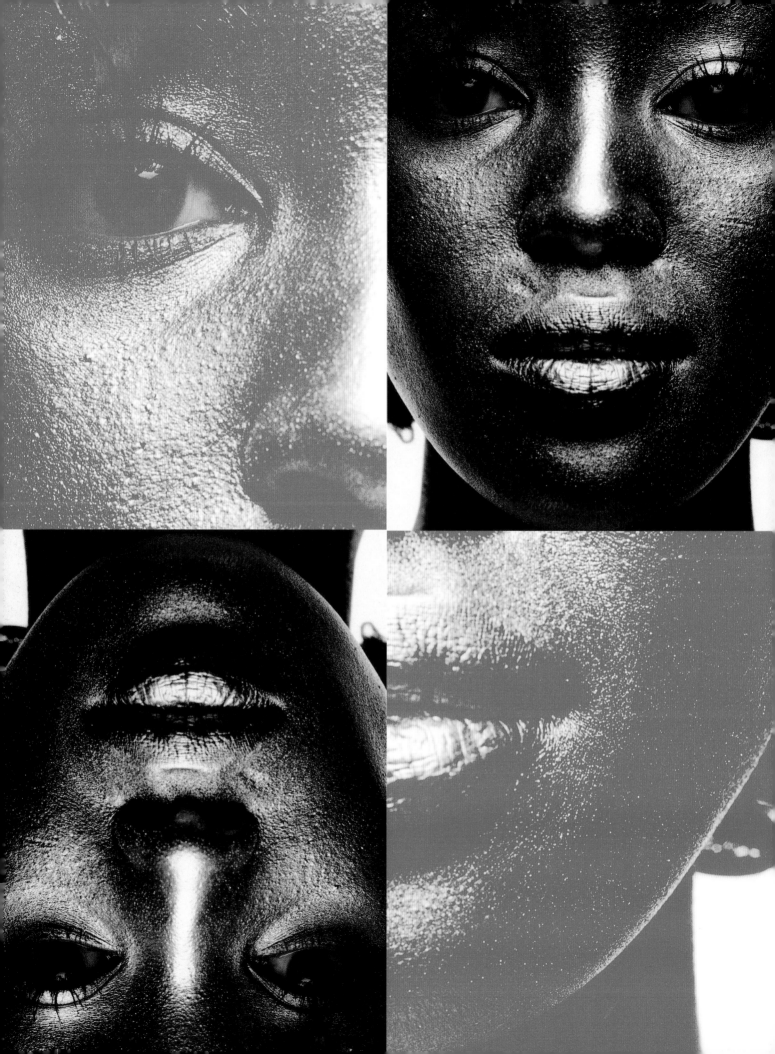

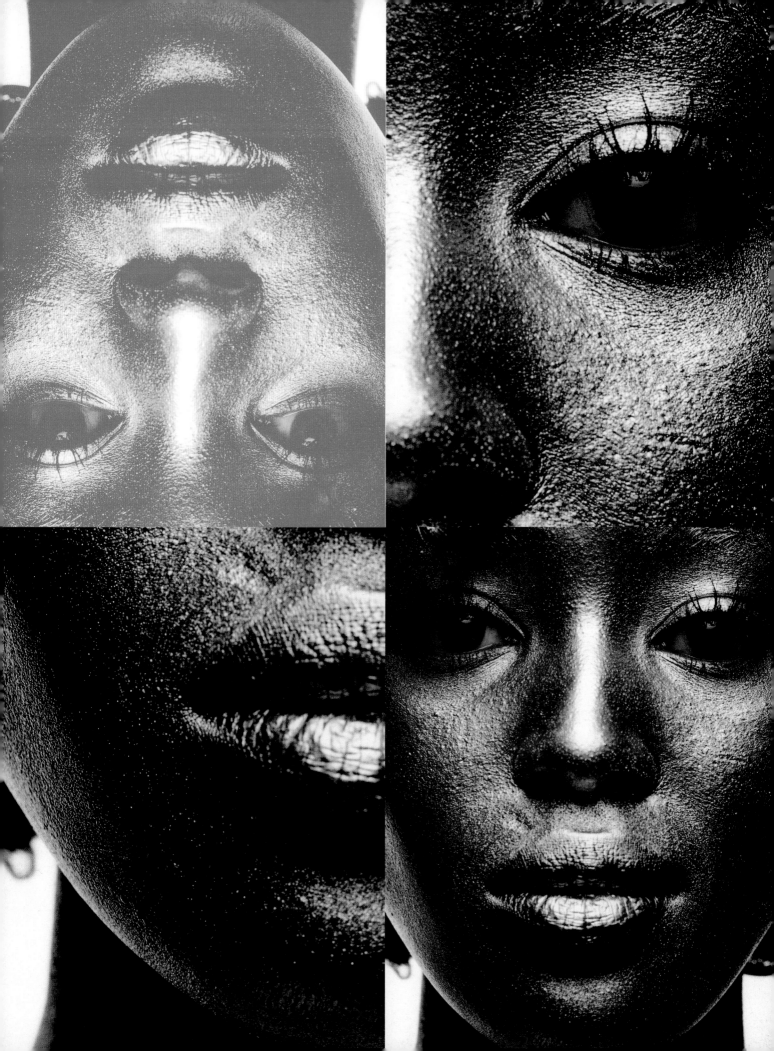

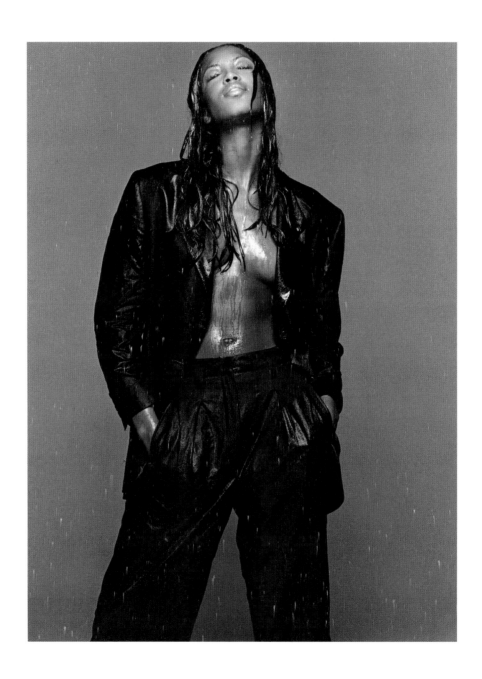

Patrick Demarchelier
New York, 1993
Harper's Bazaar

Previous spread
Thierry Le Gouès
1994
Arena

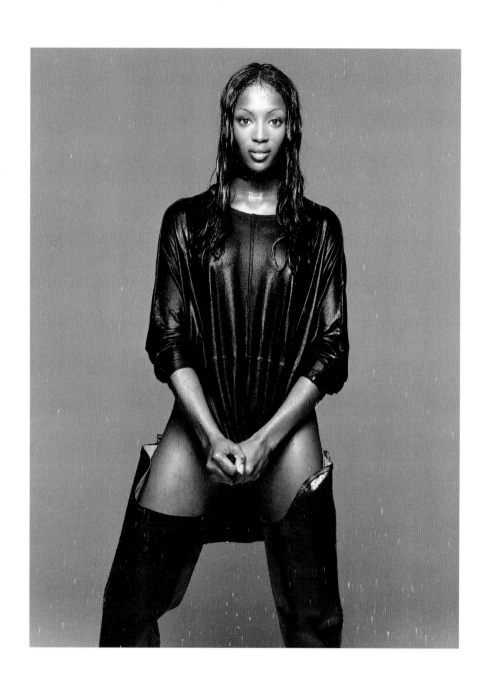

NAOMI IS CHILD TO WOMAN WRAPPED UP IN ONE. HER SMILE —INTOXICATING. HER SENSITIVITY— ALLURING. HER RANGE IS INFINITE, HER ENERGY UNIQUE. SHE'S MY FAVORITE. SHE GIVES HER ALL. —HERB RITTS

I hate to be seen as a failure in other young black girls' eyes when they read some of the stuff that's been written about me. All I can keep doing is try to break the barriers that are still there. I've been told that I'm a role model.

–Naomi, from *i-D (The Boys & Girls Issue)*, 1993

Herb Ritts
Hollywood, 1991
Interview

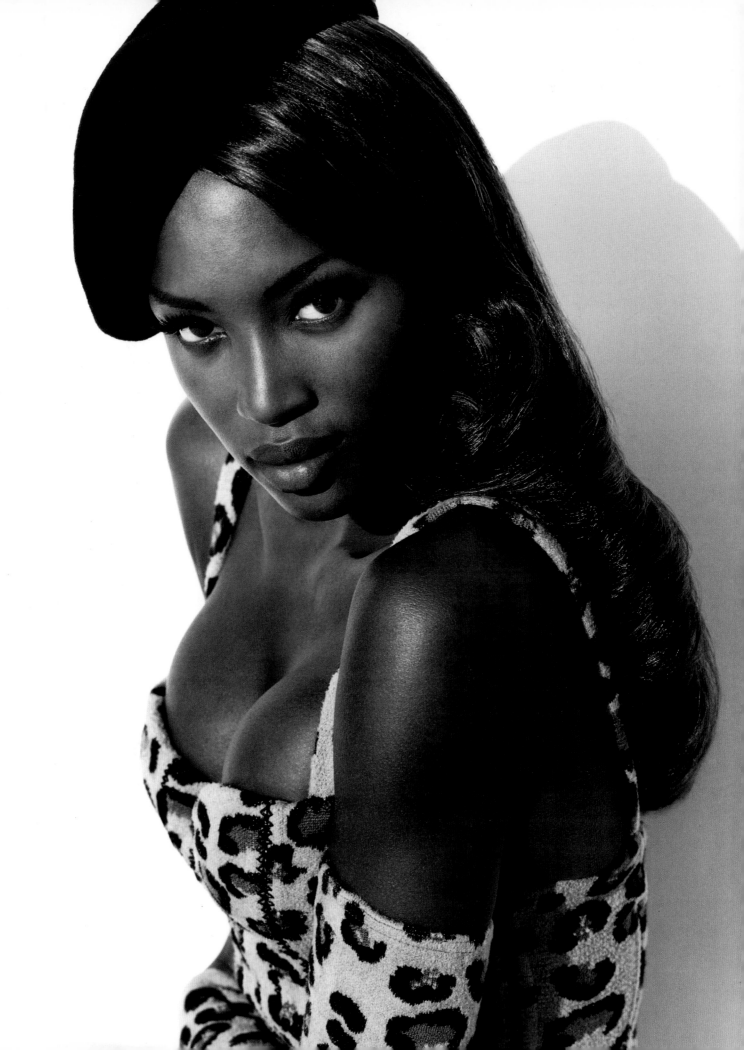

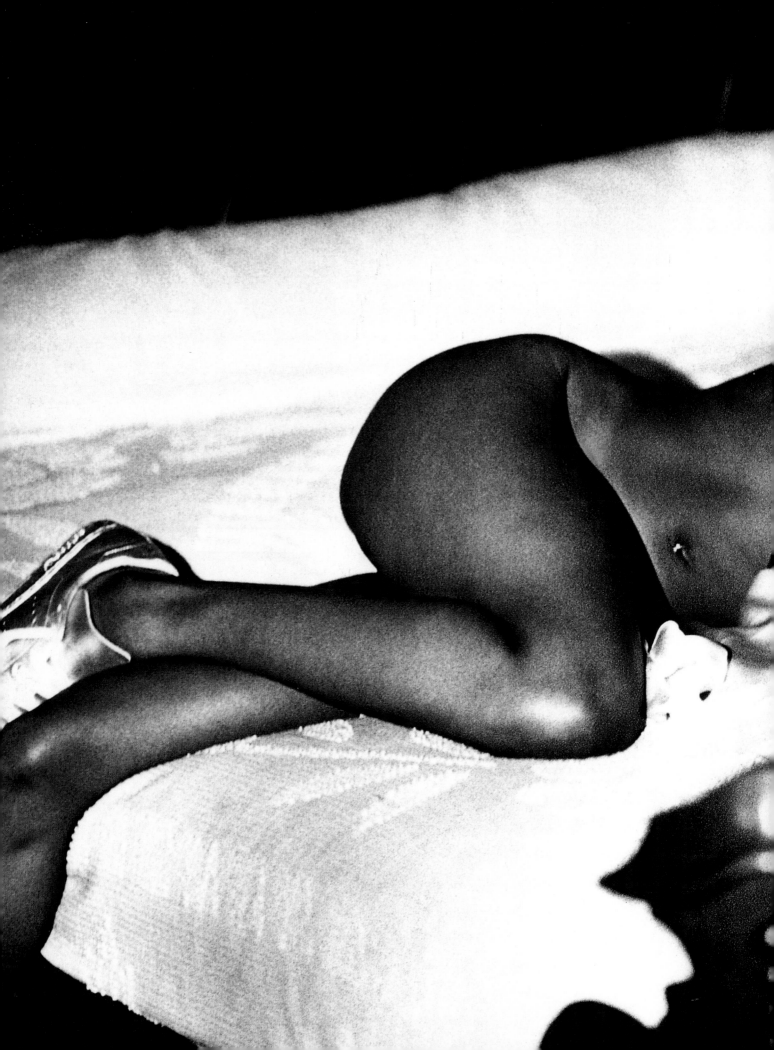

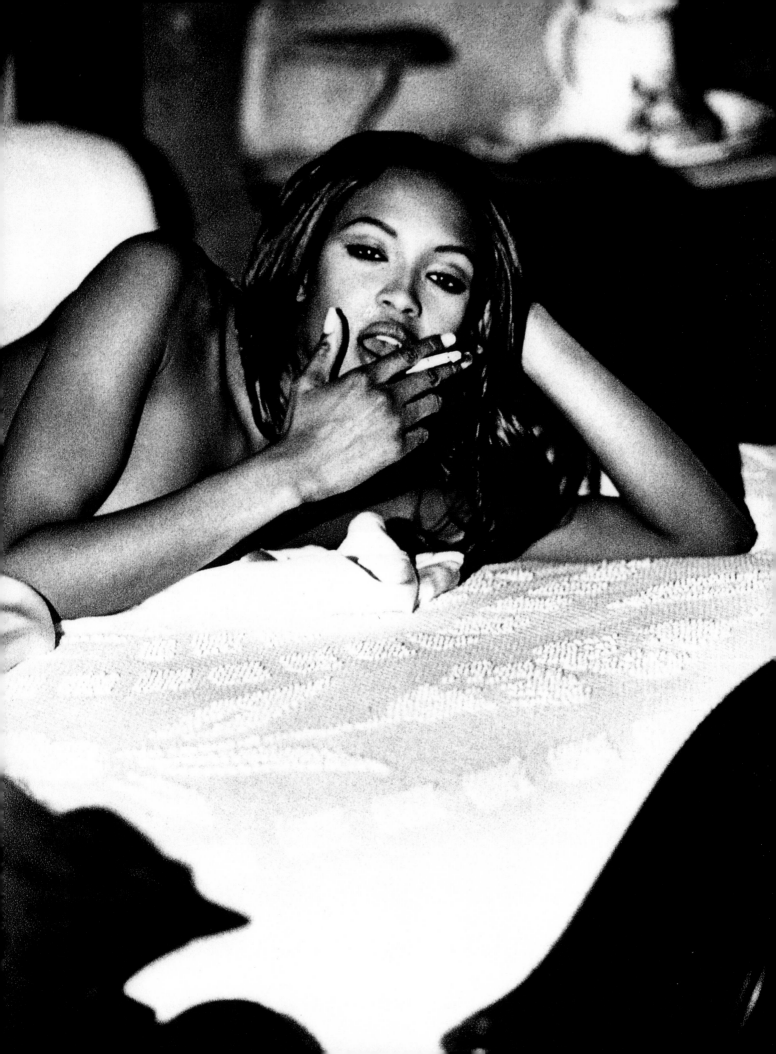

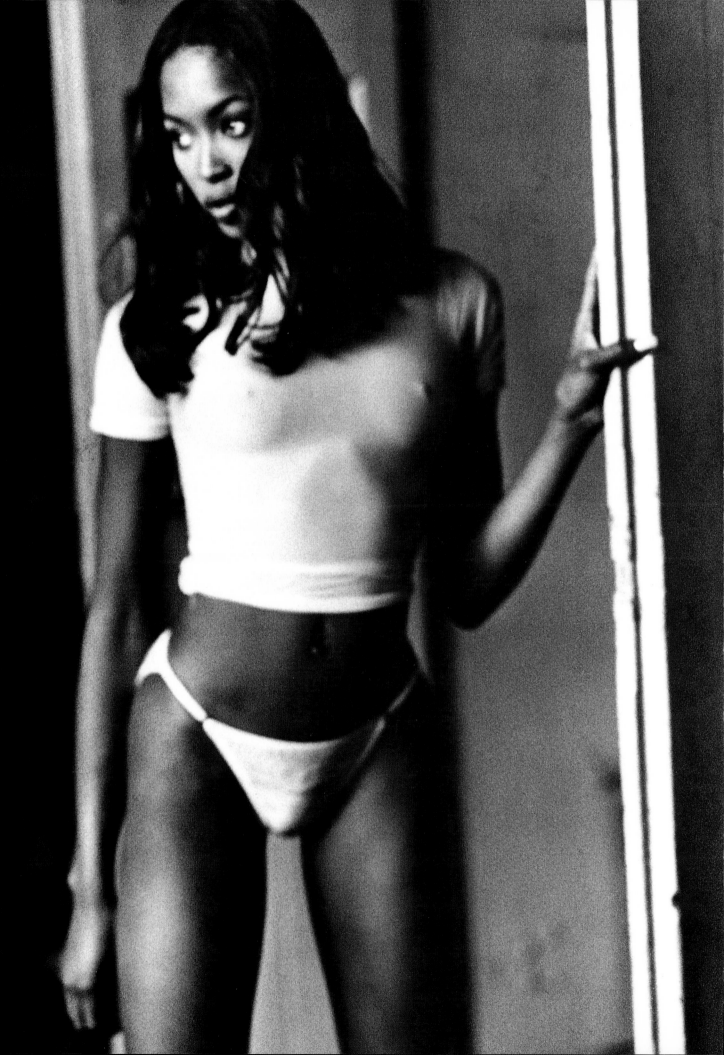

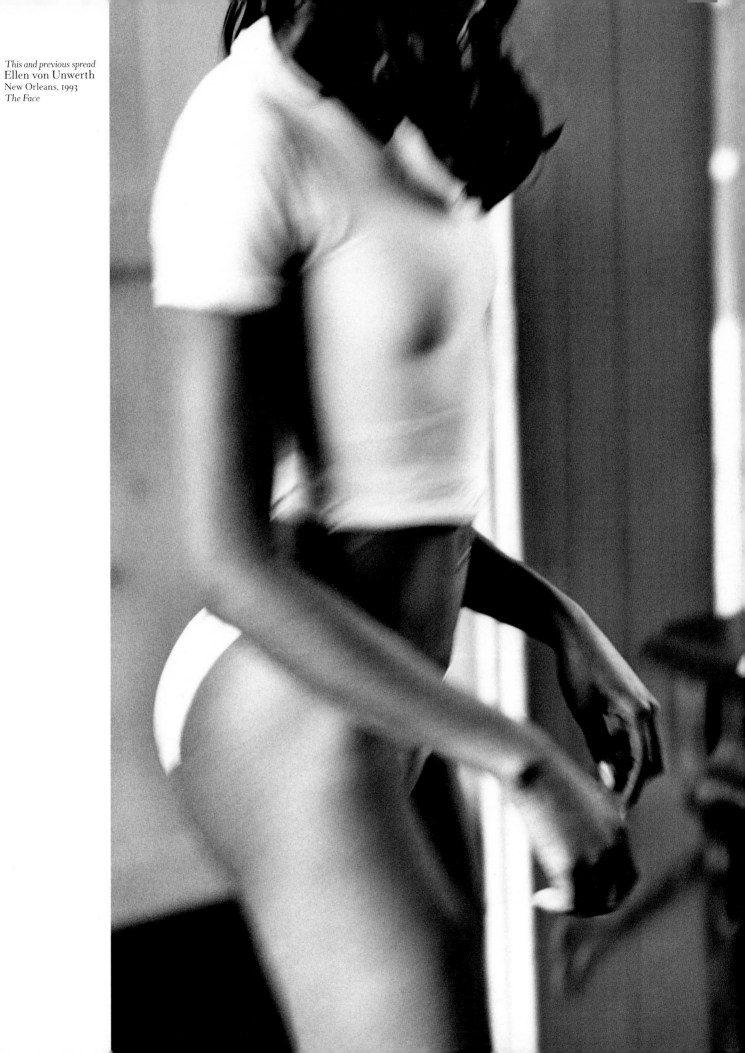

This and previous spread
Ellen von Unwerth
New Orleans, 1993
The Face

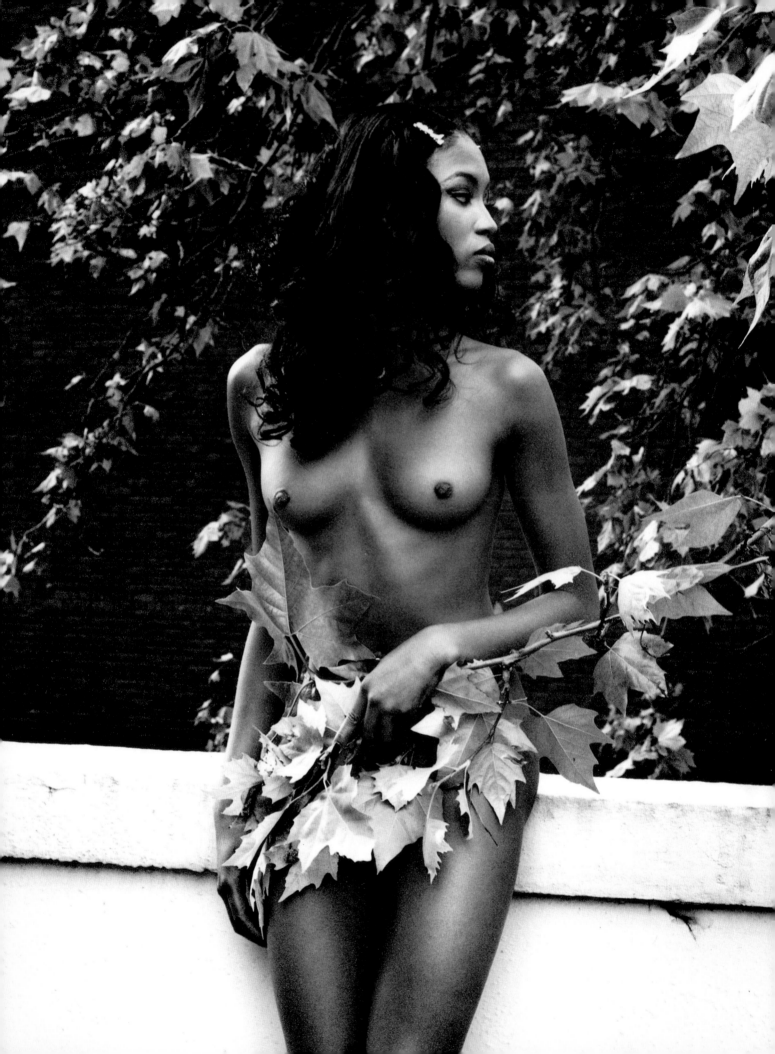

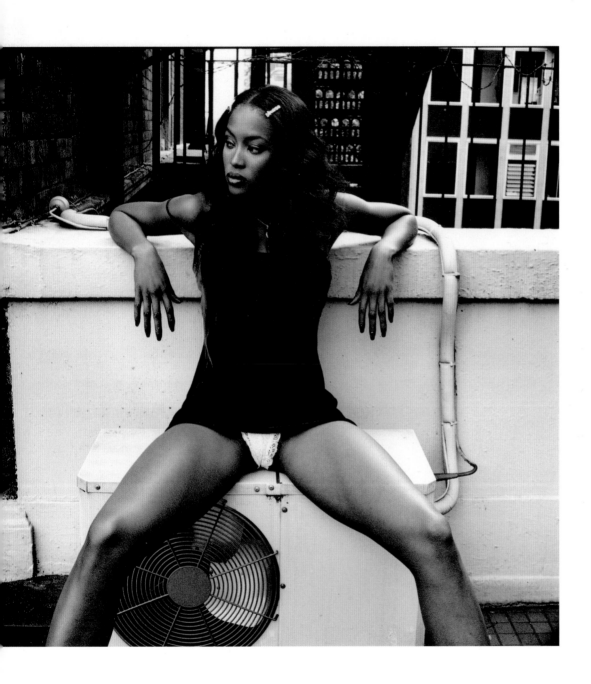

Anton Corbijn
1994 and 1995
Dutch Nieuwe Revu and *British Q*

Opposite
Anton Corbijn
1994
German Stern and *Dutch Nieuwe Revu*

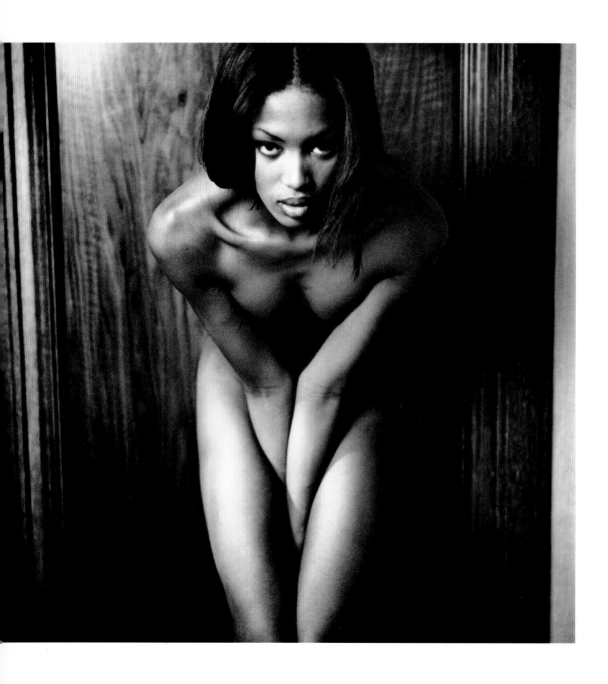

Anton Corbijn
1993 and 1996
Vogue Homme and *German Max*

Opposite
Peter Lindbergh
Jamaica, 1992
Harper's Bazaar

56

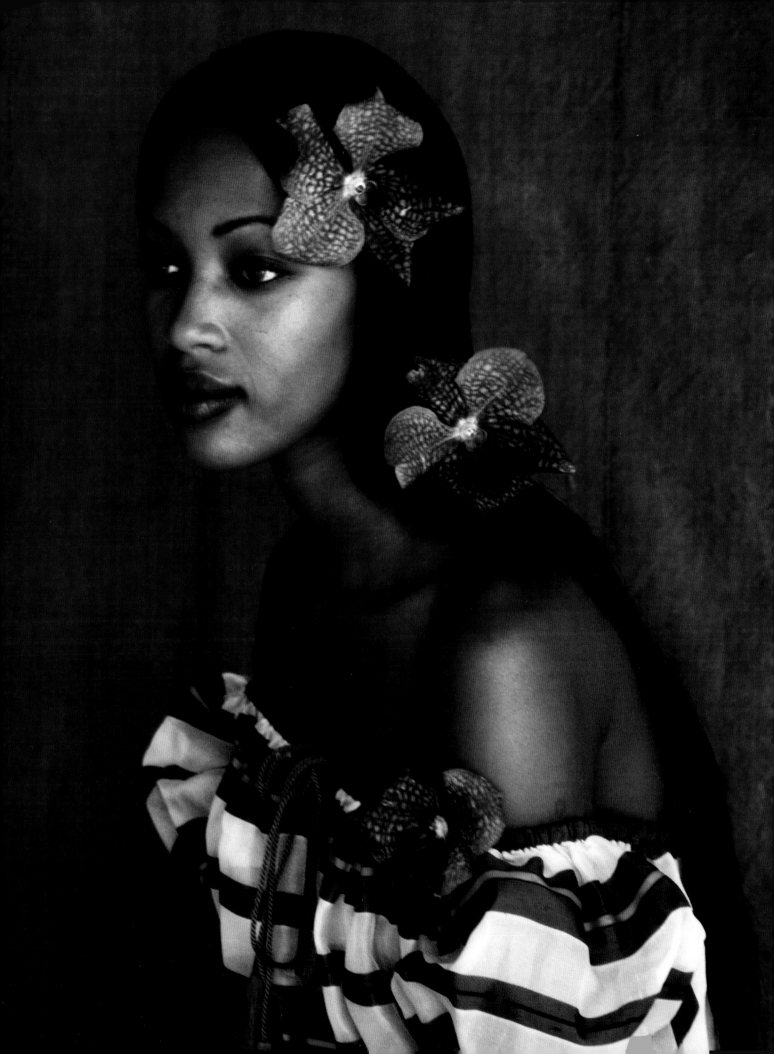

The legendary story in honor of Gauguin for HARPER'S BAZAAR was Naomi's idea. It is rather unusual that a model proposes a story to do. But Naomi is anything but a normal model. We did this story... and it was chosen as the best editorial story of that year. —Peter Lindbergh

Peter Lindbergh
Jamaica, 1992
Harper's Bazaar

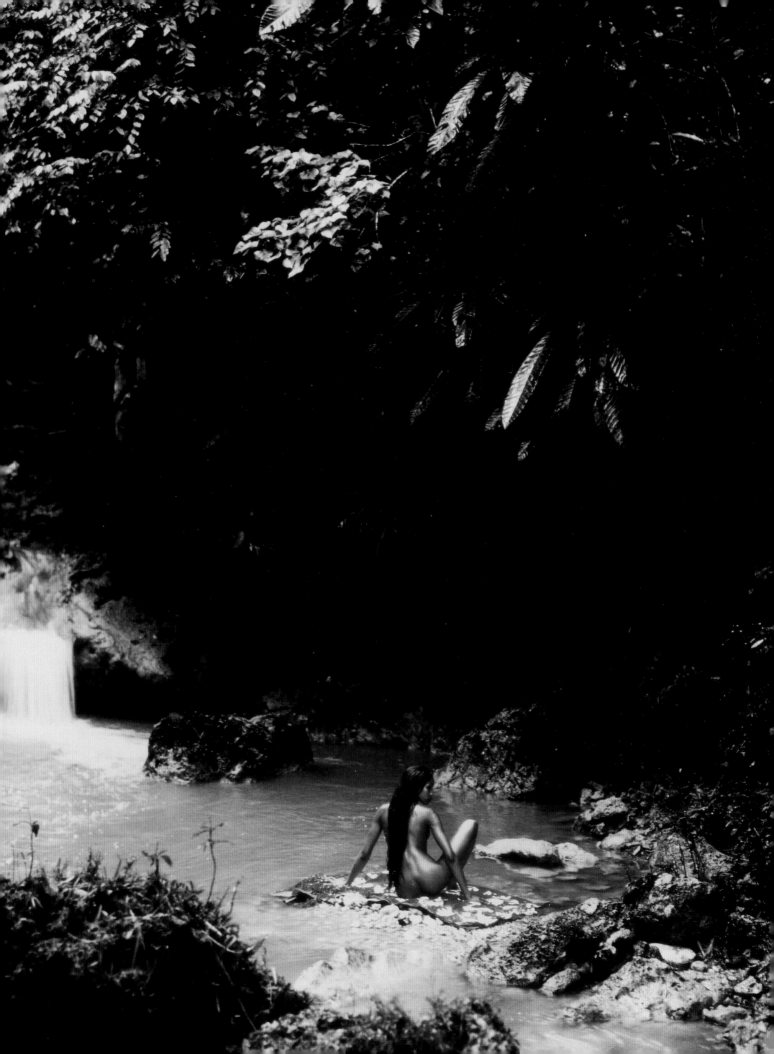

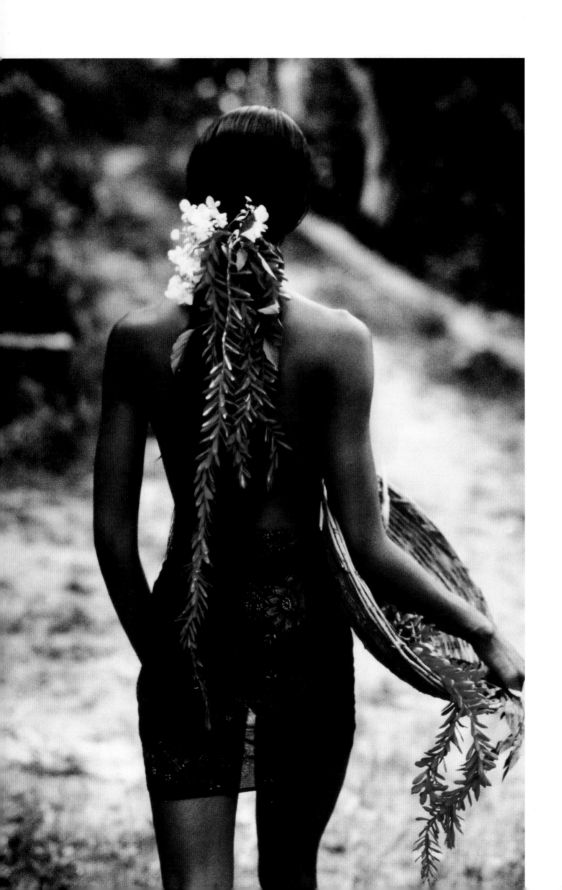

Peter Lindbergh
Jamaica, 1992
Harper's Bazaar

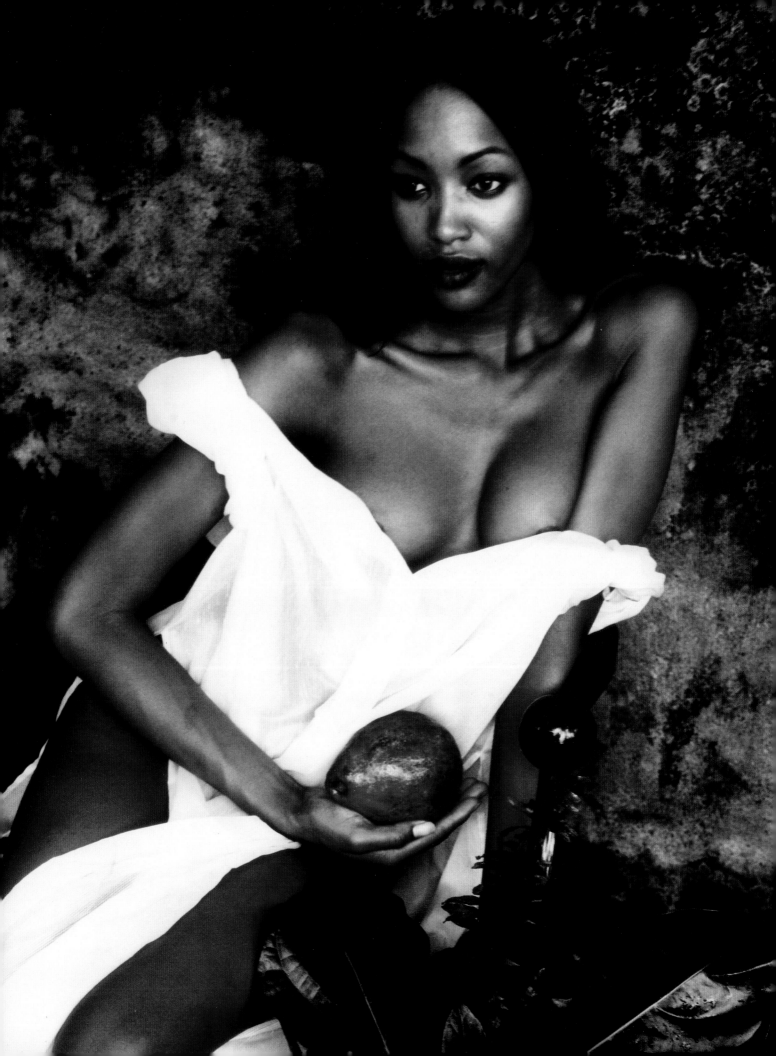

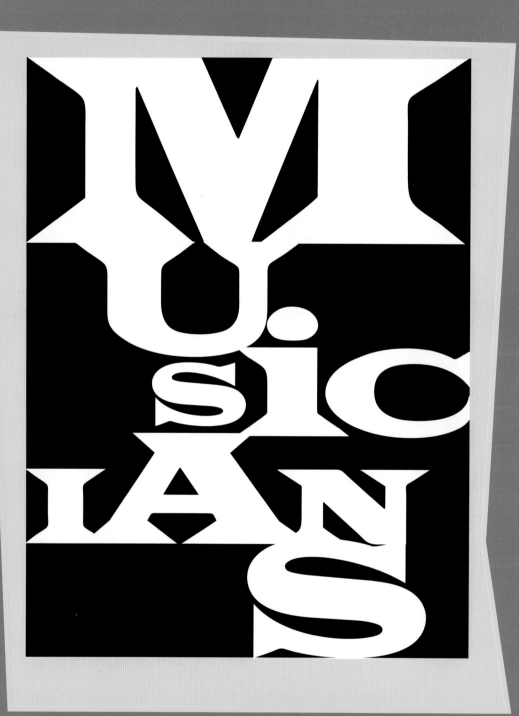

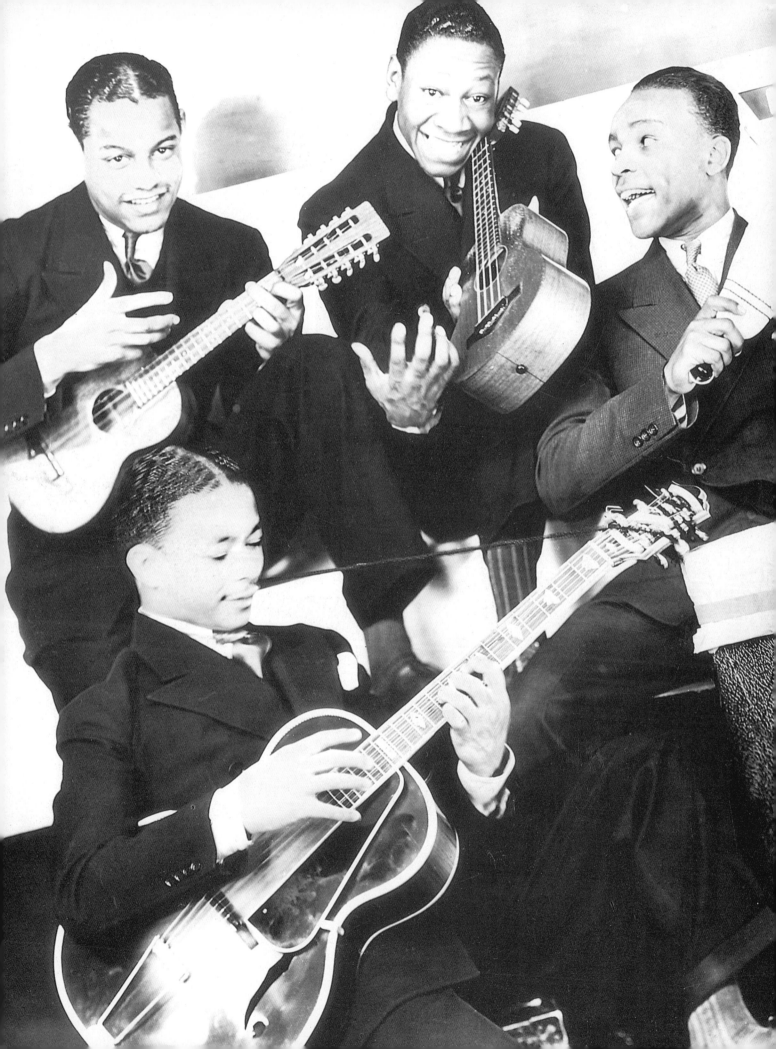

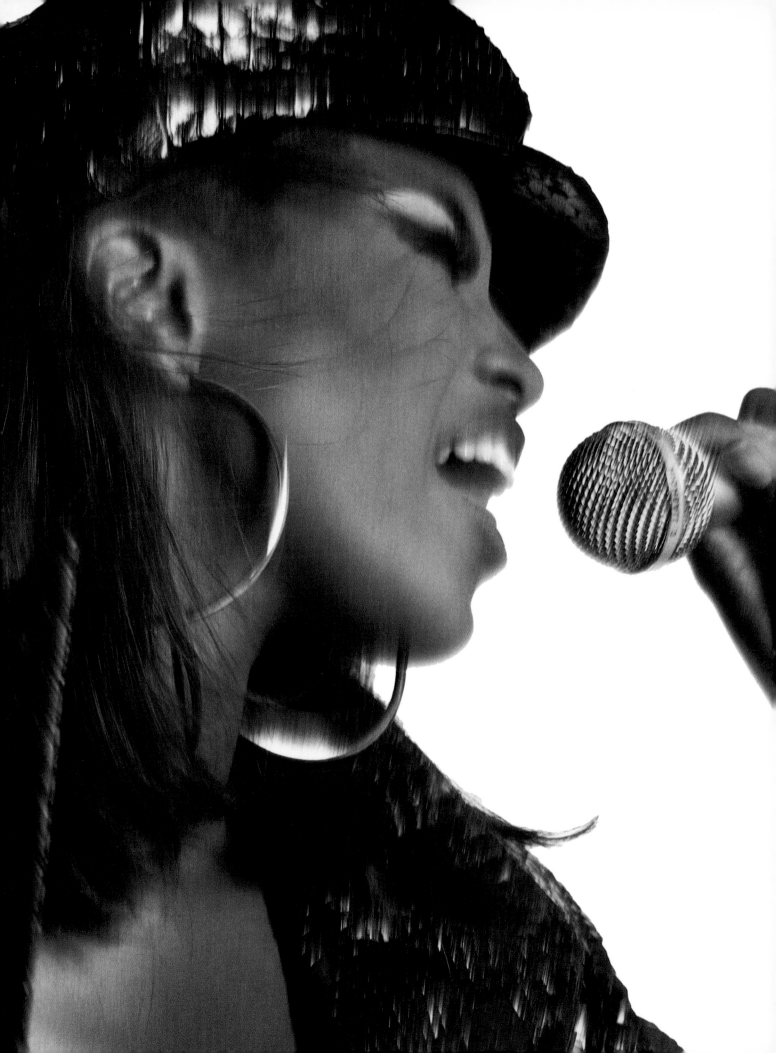

"I don't really know how to write songs,

I can just write poems. And I don't care if this

is the one and only record [*Babywoman*] I ever do, just so long as I tried it."

—Naomi, from *i-D (The Boys & Girls Issue)*, 1993

Steven Meisel
1989
Italian Vogue

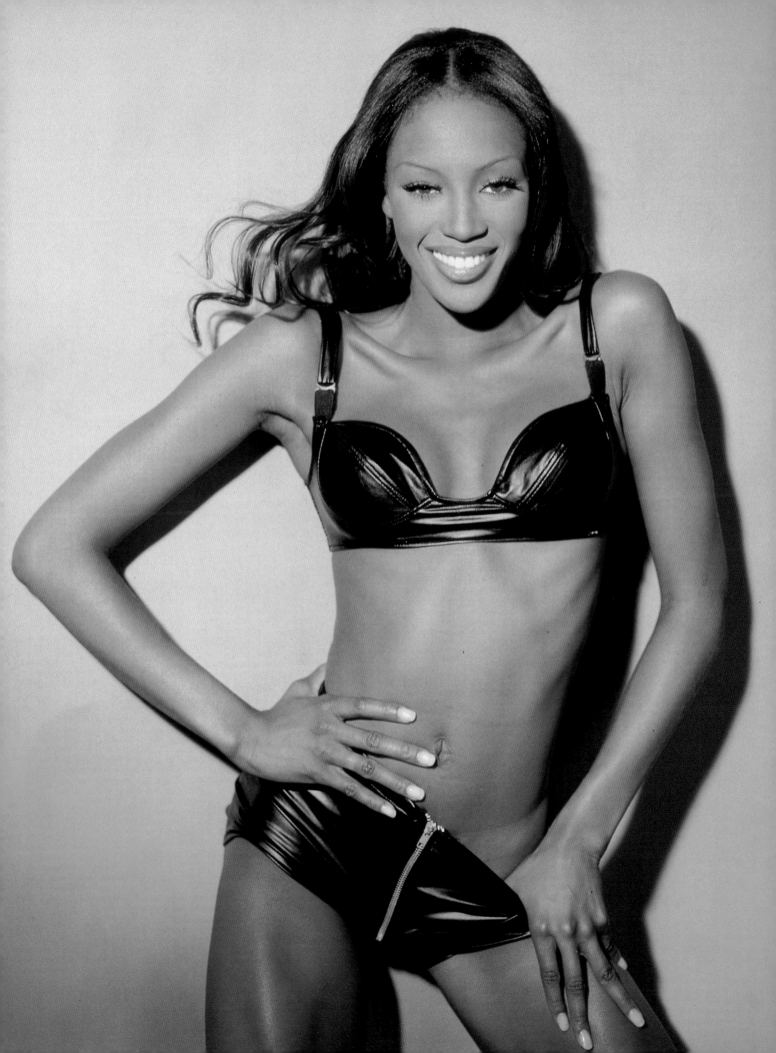

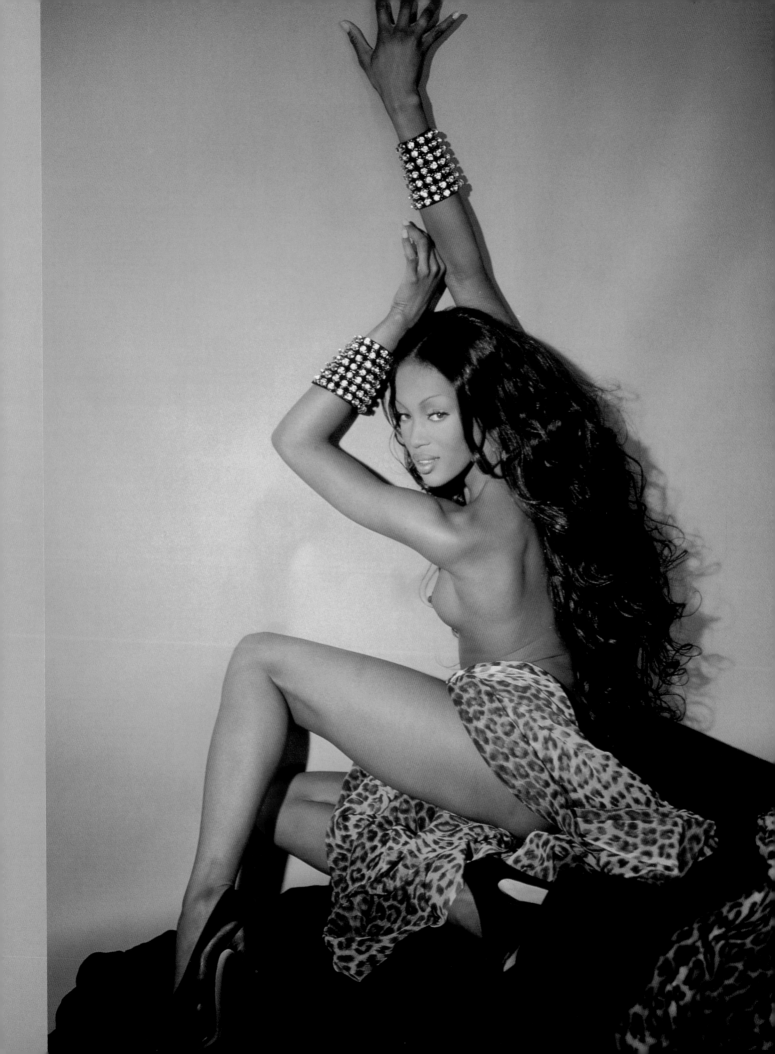

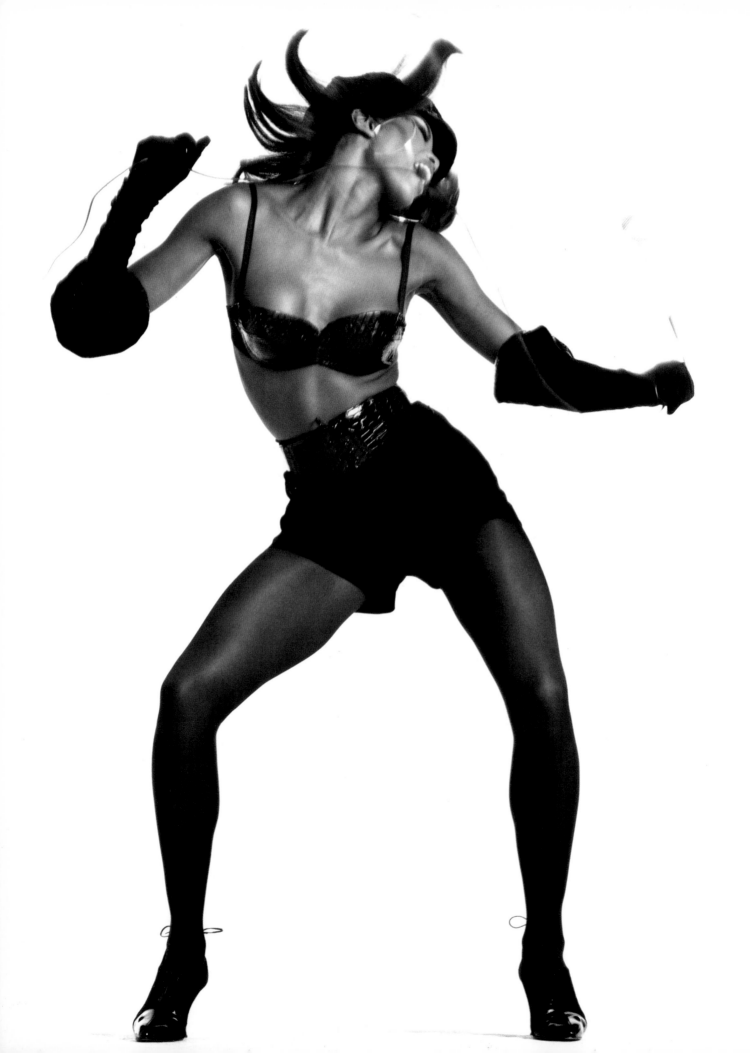

SHE IS ONE OF THE MOST BEAUTIFUL WOMEN I'VE

EVER HAD THE PLEASURE OF MEETING AND

AND I'VE HAD THE PLEASURE OF MEETING HER FAMILY,

KNOWING—AND I'M NOT JUST TALKING PHYSICALLY.

AND LET ME TELL YOU... THEY'RE ALL BEAUTIFUL.

SHE HAS SUCH ATTITUDE—IN A POSITIVE SENSE—

I DON'T KNOW IF IT'S THE GENES OR IF THEY ALL JUST EAT

SHE'S GOT THE BEST WALK I'VE SEEN. NAOMI DON'T

"PRETTY FOOD," BUT THEY ARE SOMETHING ELSE.

JUST WALK THAT RUNWAY, SHE STRUTS. WHEN

AND LIKE NAOMI THEY'RE ALL JUST SWEET, PERSONAL,

I SEE HER DO HER THING, I JUST SAY TO MYSELF

FRIENDLY, AND DOWN TO EARTH PEOPLE...

"WALK ON GIRL, GO AHEAD WITH YOUR BAD SELF."

—PATTI LABELLE

Previous spread
Sante D'Orazio
New York, 1992
British Vogue

Opposite
Steven Meisel
1989
Italian Vogue

Following spread
Paolo Roversi
Paris, 1992
Jimi Hendrix, unpublished

If you're going to get into this business, stay balanced and in contact with your family. Soon as something happens, Mum is the first one I call.

—Naomi, from *Arthur Elgort's Models Manual*

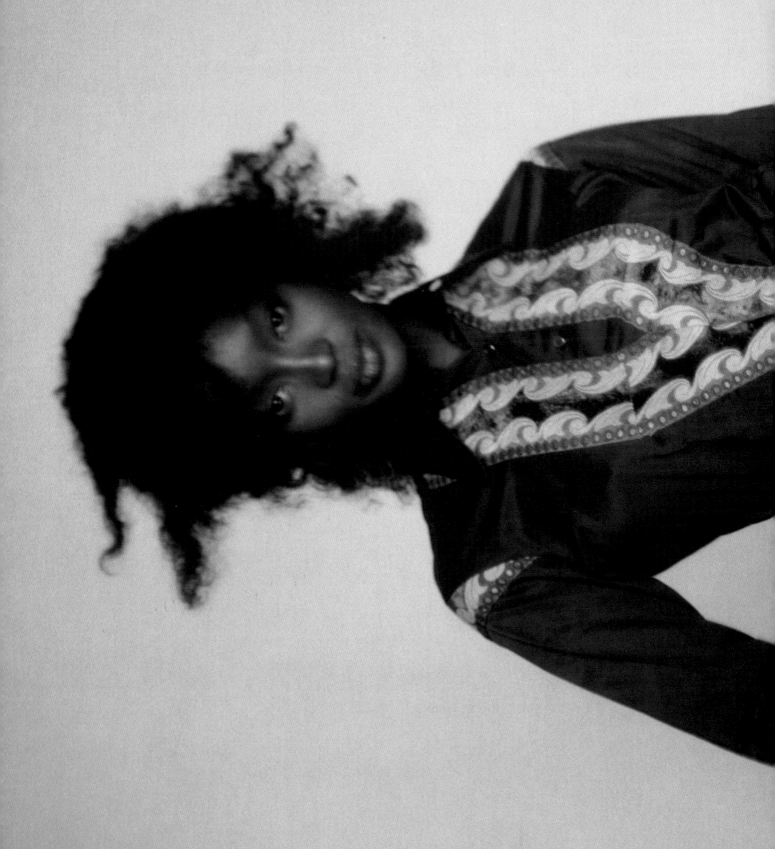

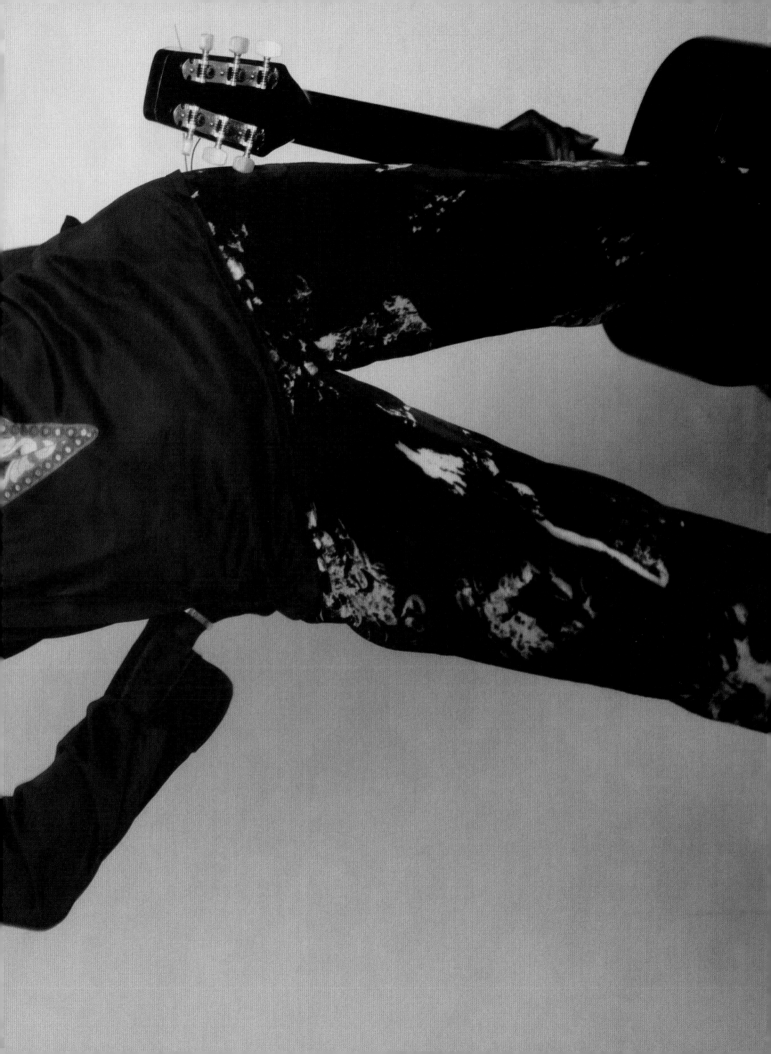

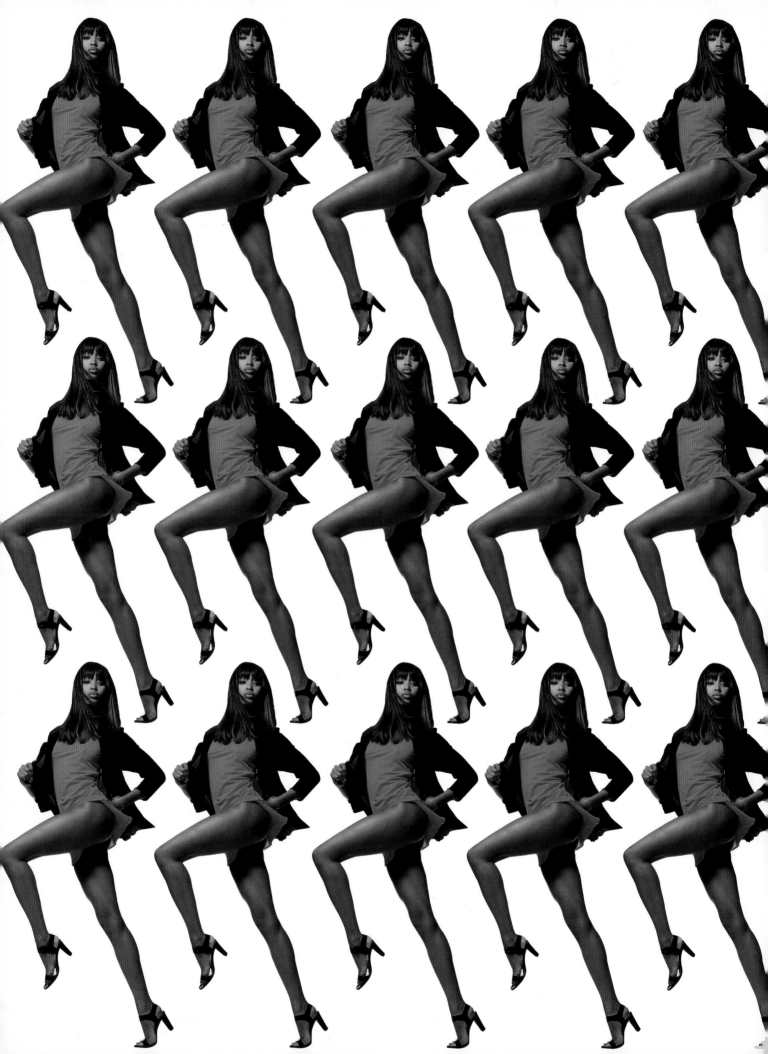

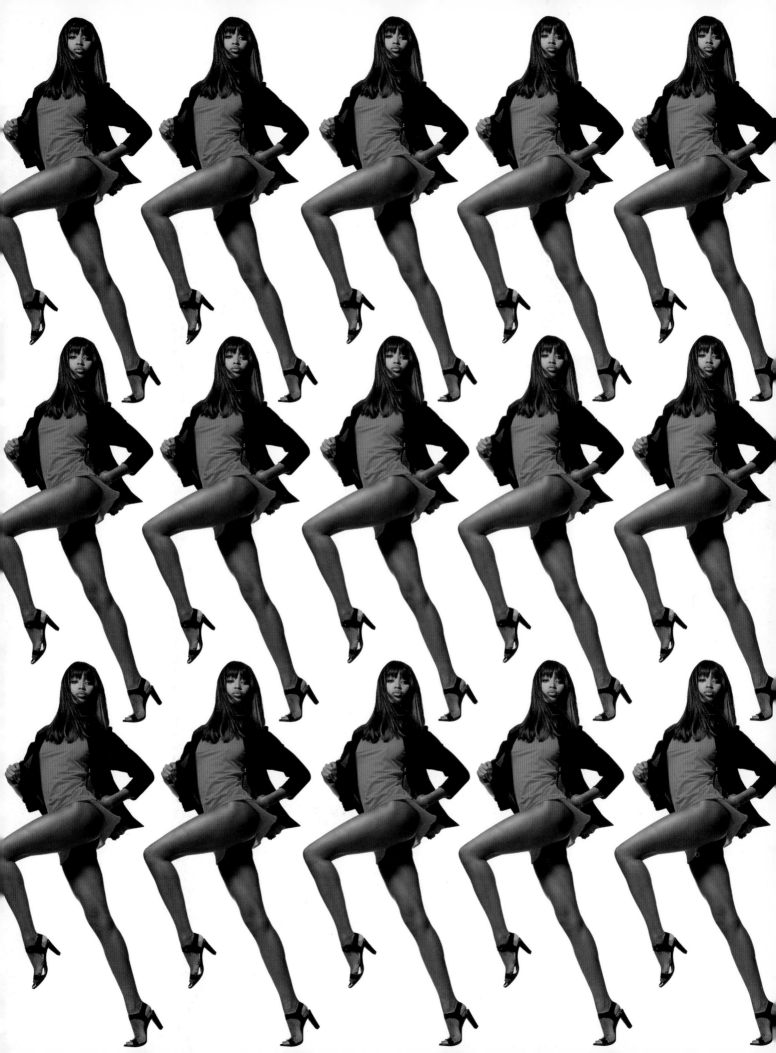

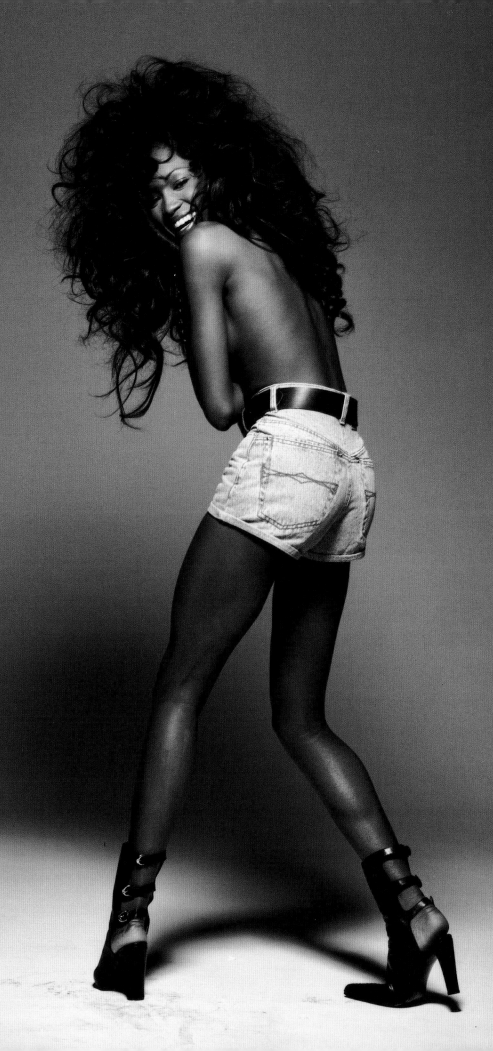

Previous spread
Albert Watson
New York, 1994
British Vogue

This spread
Michael Williams
New York, 1992
Falmer Jeans campaign, U.K.

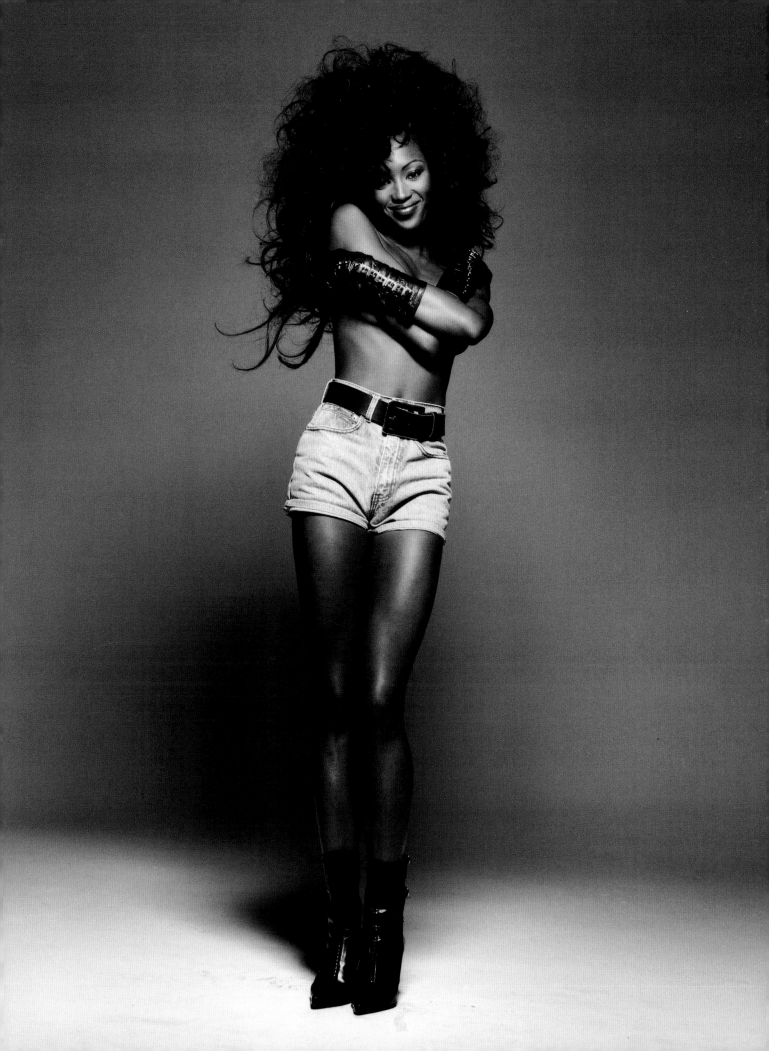

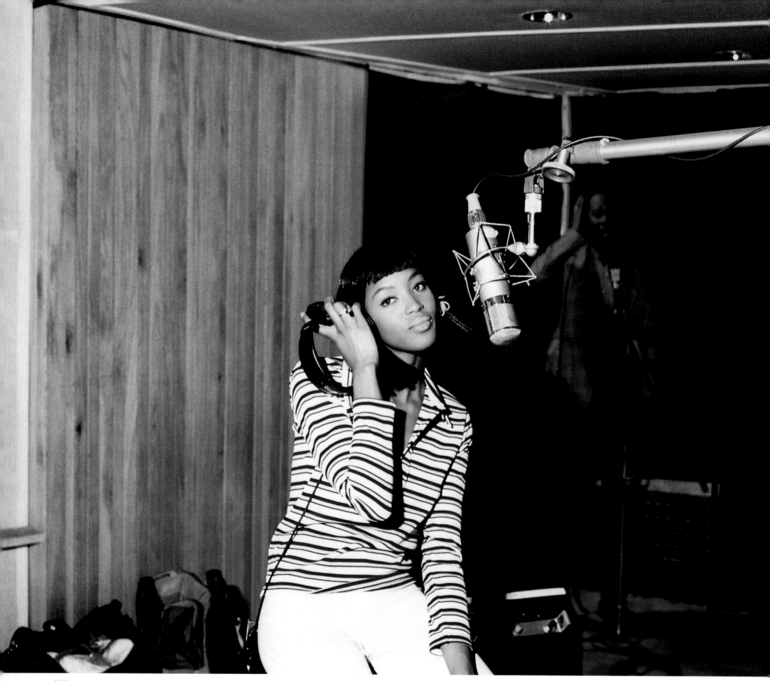

I'M
TIRED
OF
ALL
THE
FUSS
ABOUT
MODELS
BEING
OVERPAID.
JUST
GO
TO
A
FASHION
SHOW
AND
WATCH
NAOMI
CAMPBELL
PROWL
DOWN
THE
RUNWAY
AND
YOU'LL
REALIZE
THAT
SHE'S
WORTH
EVERY
PENNY.
EVERY
TIME
I
SEE
HER
IN
PERSON,
HER
BEAUTY
ASTOUNDS
ME.
**—ELTON
JOHN**

I'm just another average girl that admires you a lot...you are my biggest role model (and by that I certainly do not mean the fattest!)

—from a fan letter

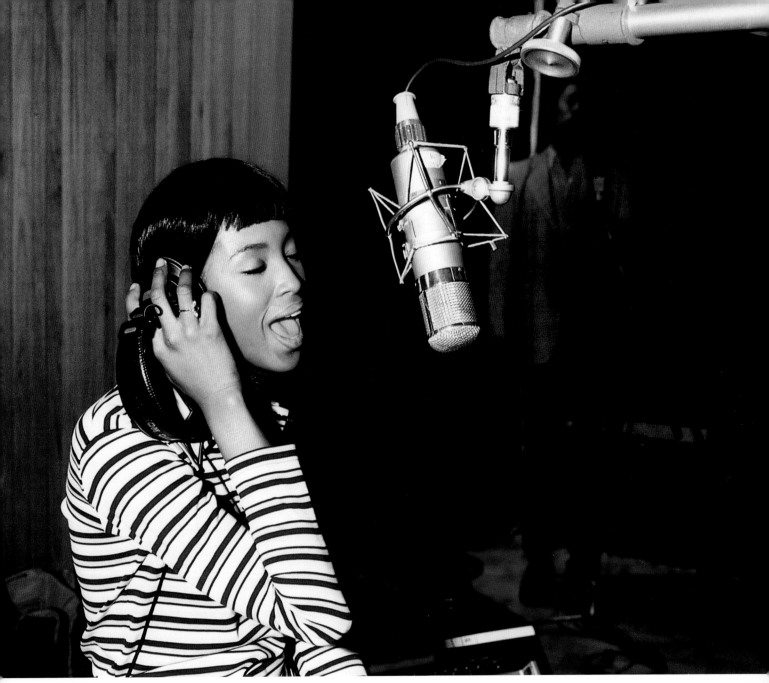

NAOMI
IS
A
STUNNINGLY
BEAUTIFUL
GIRL,
VERY
TOUGH,
VERY
AMBITIOUS,
BUT
WITH
A
HEART
OF
SOLID
GOLD,

A
GOOD
FRIEND.
—ERIC
CLAPTON

Jack Pierson
New York, 1994
unpublished

Following spread
Ellen von Unwerth
1991
Italian Vogue

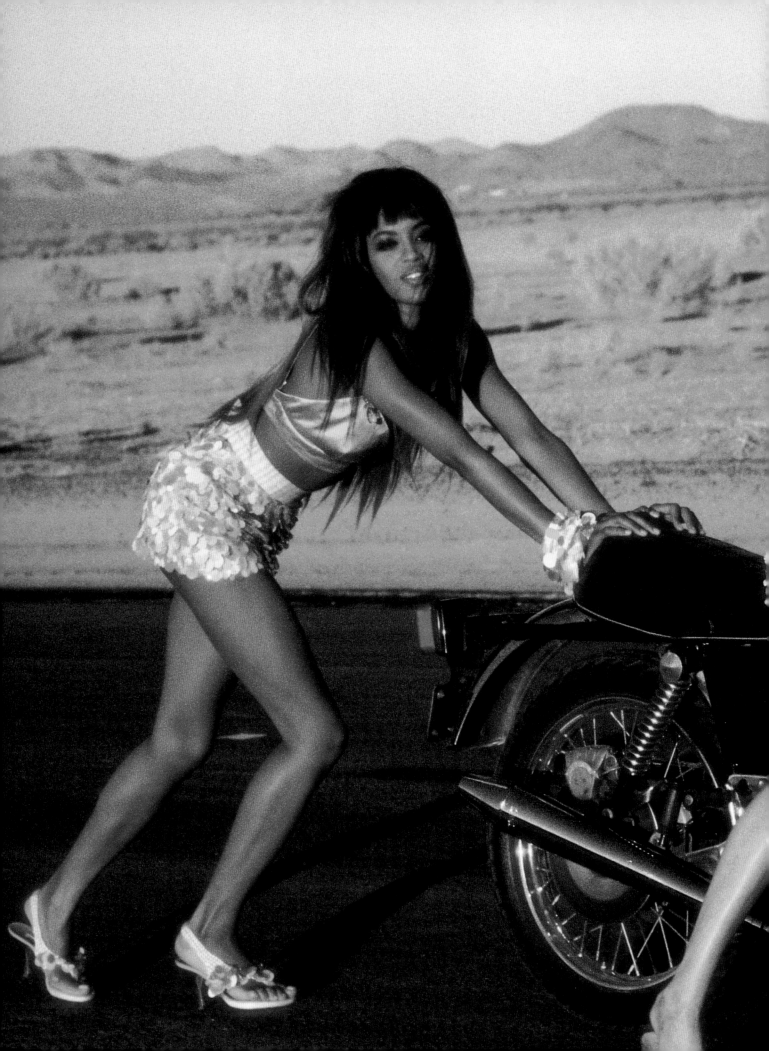

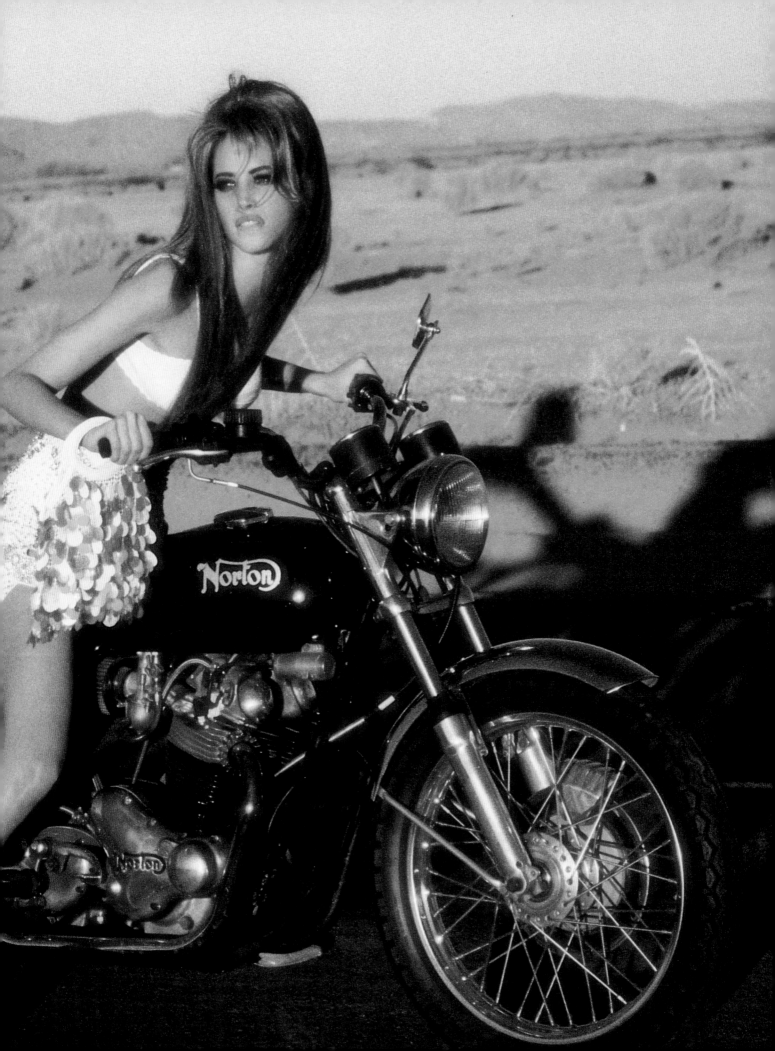

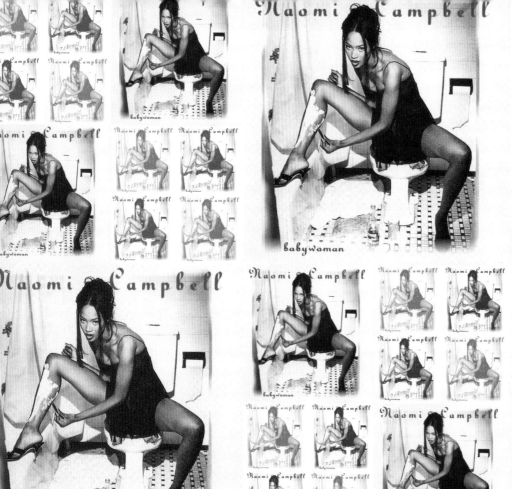
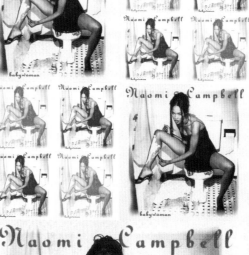
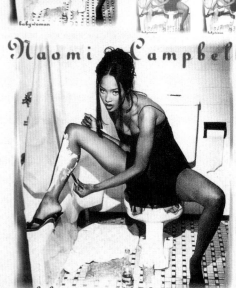
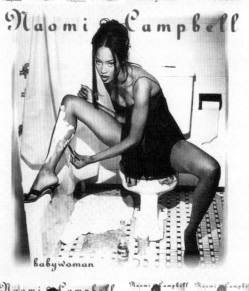
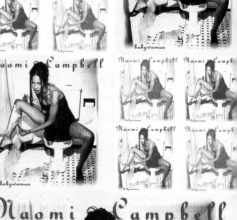
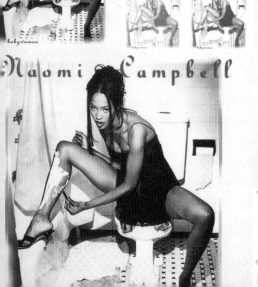
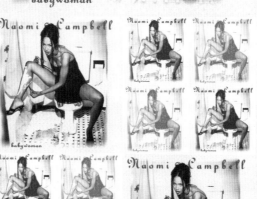
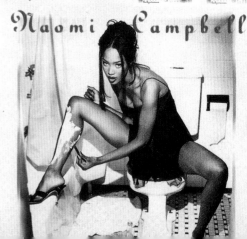

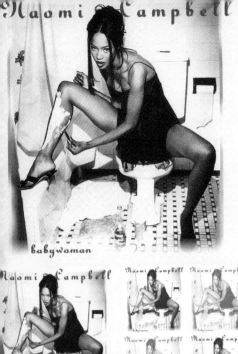
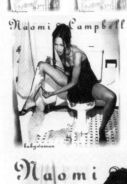
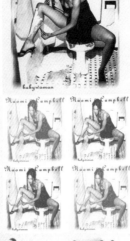
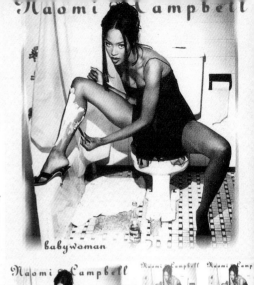
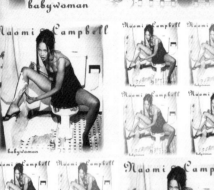
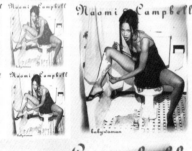
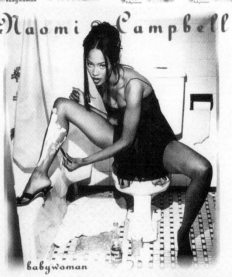
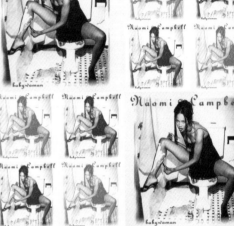
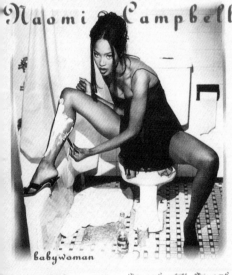
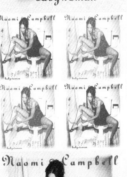
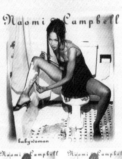
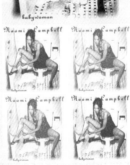
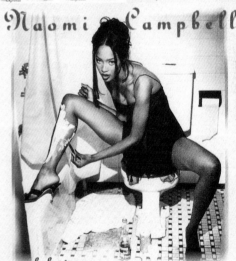

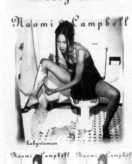
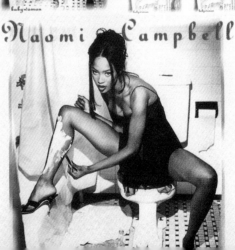
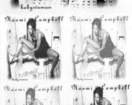
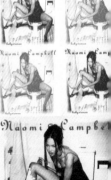

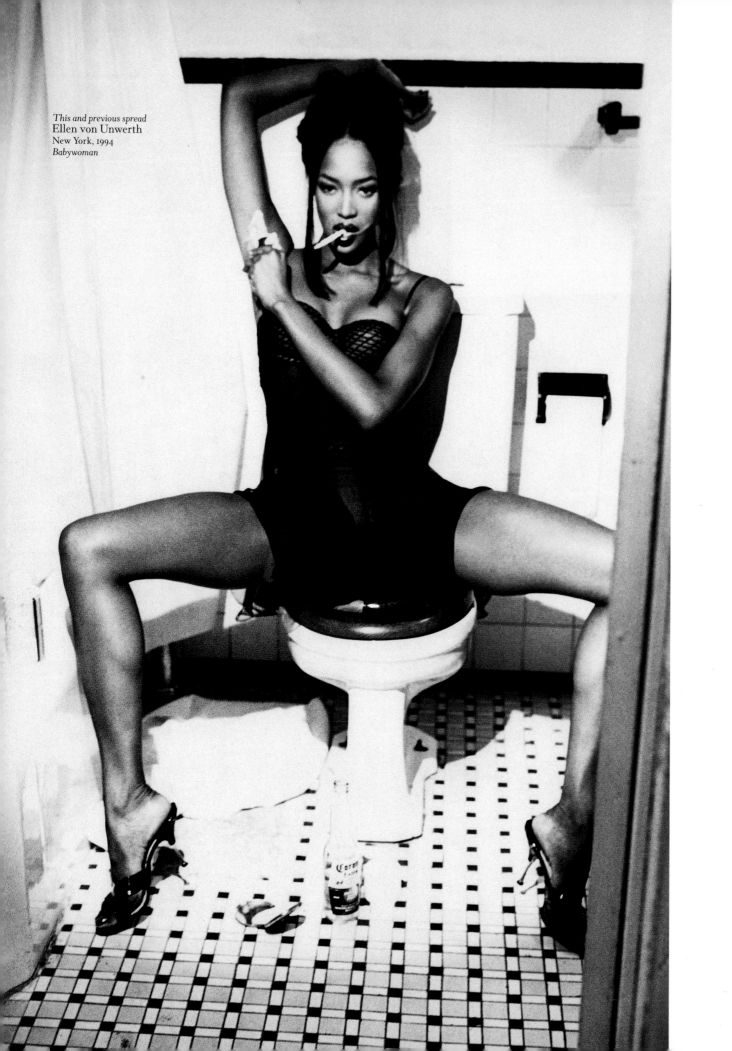

This and previous spread
Ellen von Unwerth
New York, 1994
Babywoman

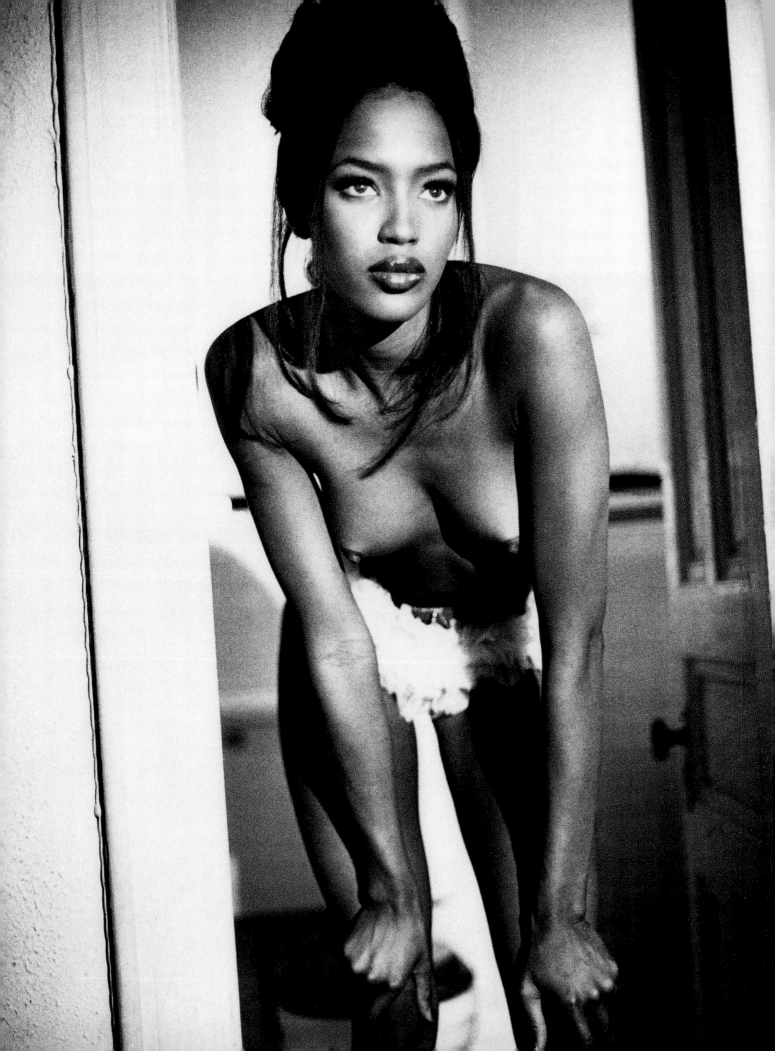

NAOMI, GENEROUS TO A FAULT GENEROUS WITH HER FAULTS... WIDE OPEN, AKIMBO, MISCHIEVOUS AND MYSTERIOUS, A SILENT MOVIE STAR IN AN AGE OF NOISE, BEYOND

BLACK AND WHITE BEYOND COLOR... BUT DIFFERENT FROM THAT GOLDEN AGE OF HOLLYWOOD IN THAT NAOMI IS IN CHARGE OF EVERYTHING... EXCEPT HER HEART. —BONO

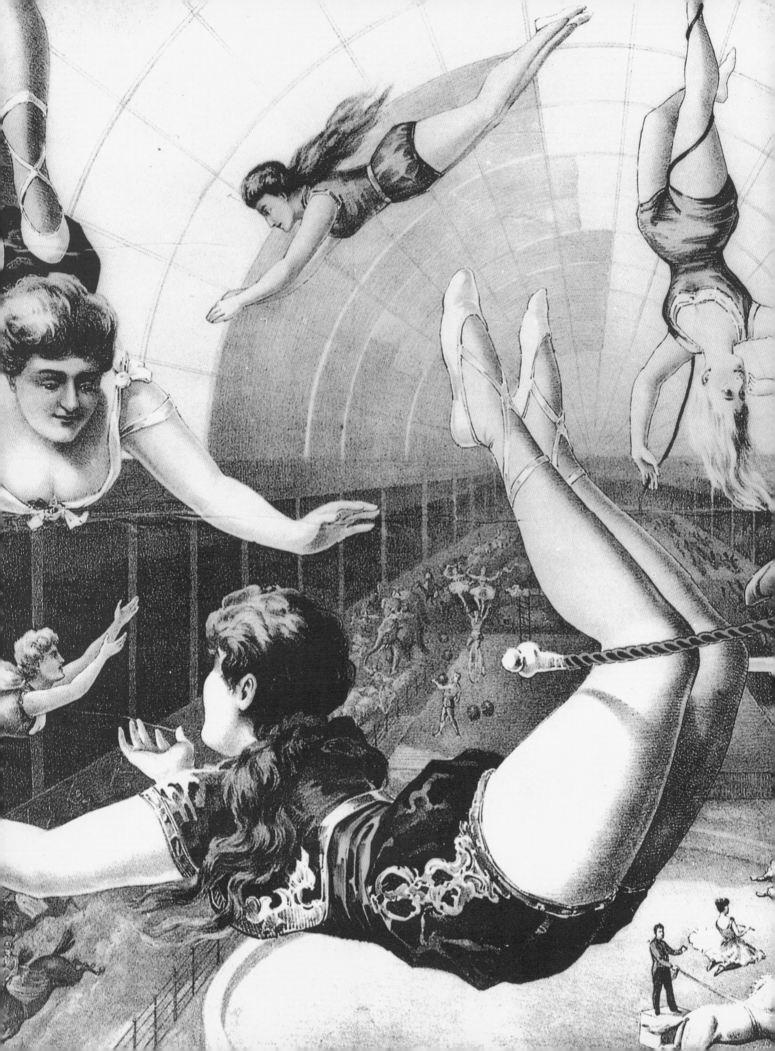

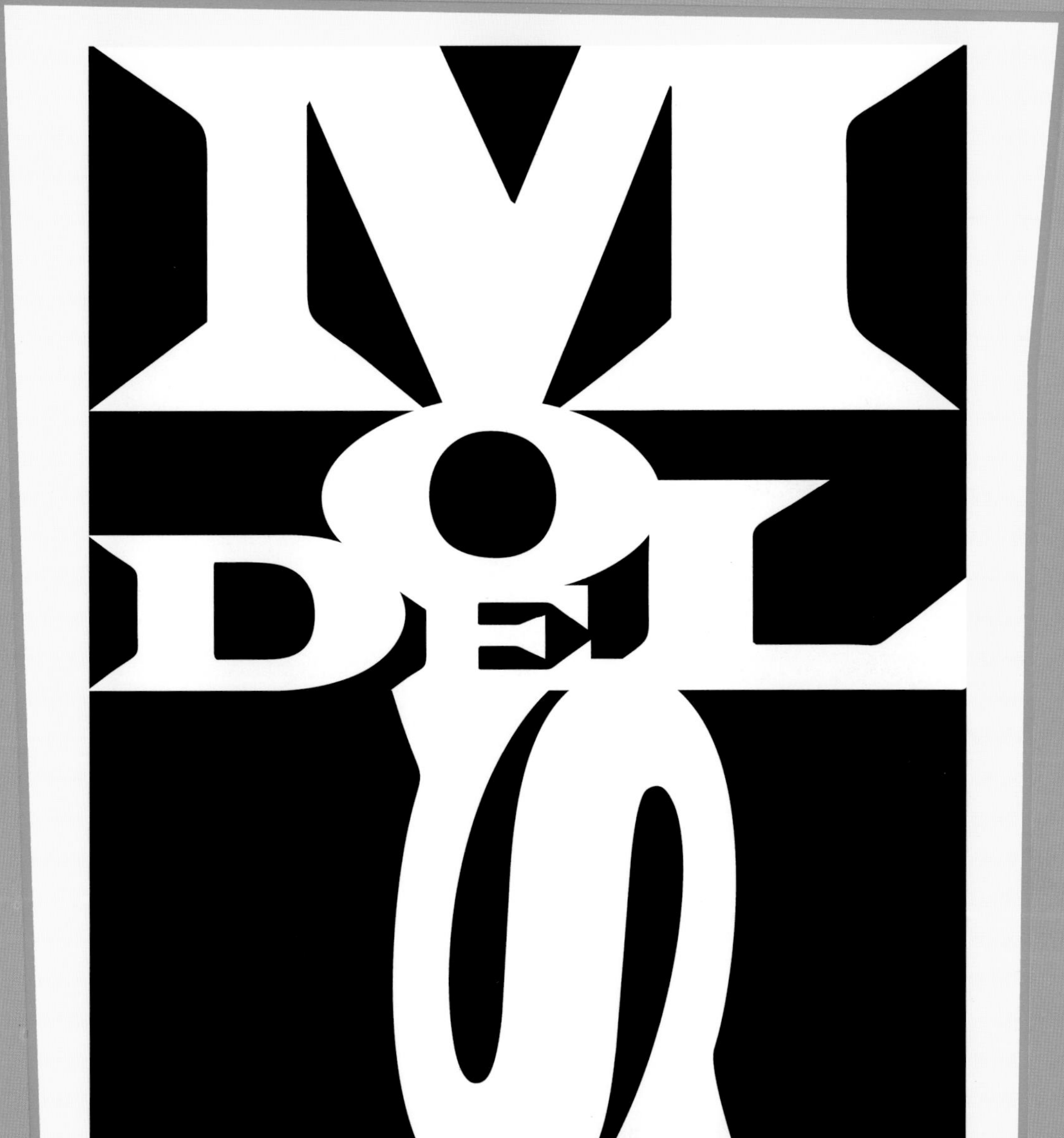
M
O
DEL

"Modeling is a merciless business. You need to construct
some protection and you get called a bitch for it. . . .
You can't just be walked over and taken advantage of.
You have to have some barriers."

—Naomi, from *You*, 1995

Thierry Le Gouès
1994
unpublished

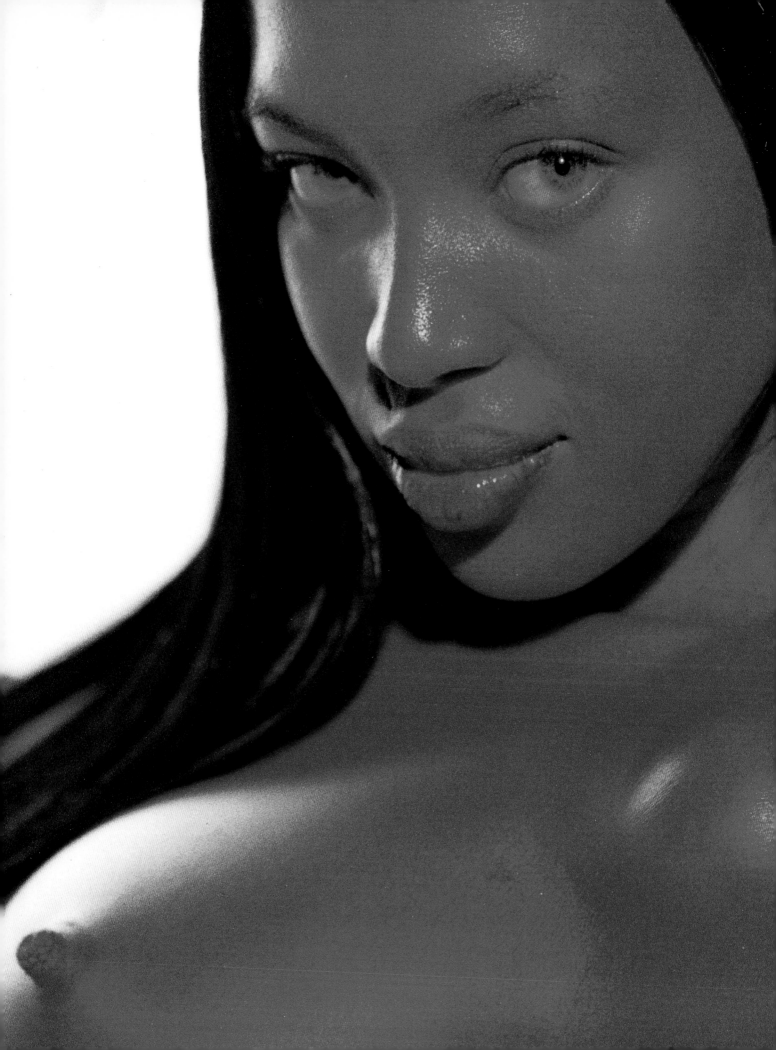

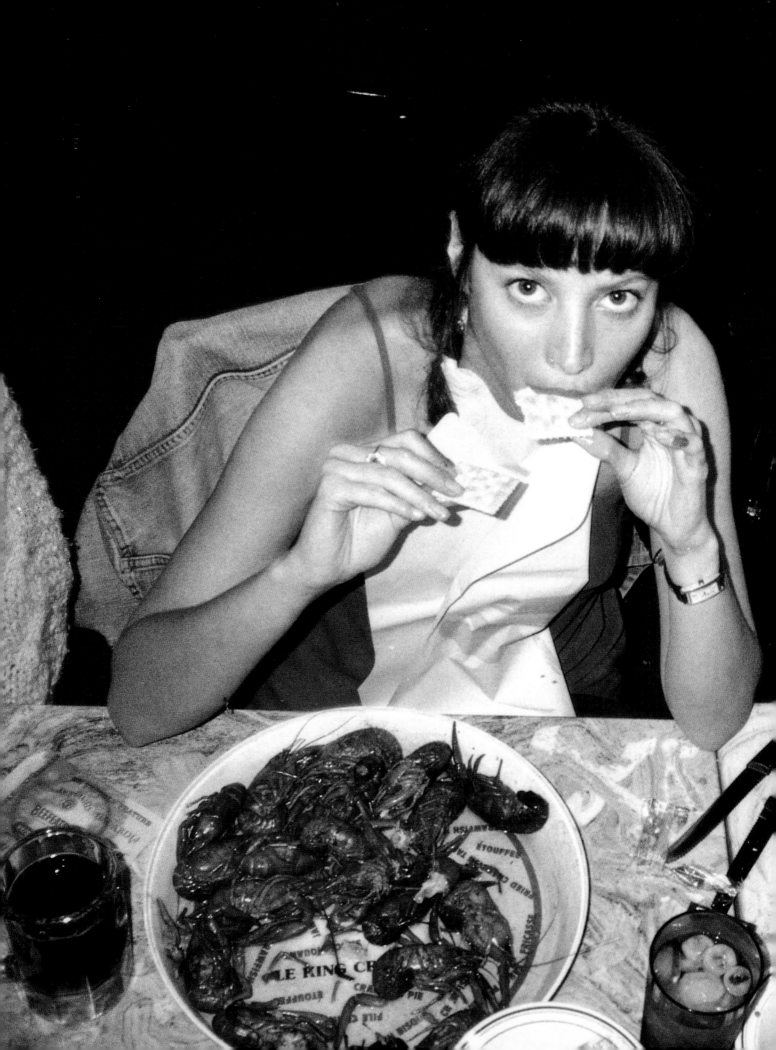

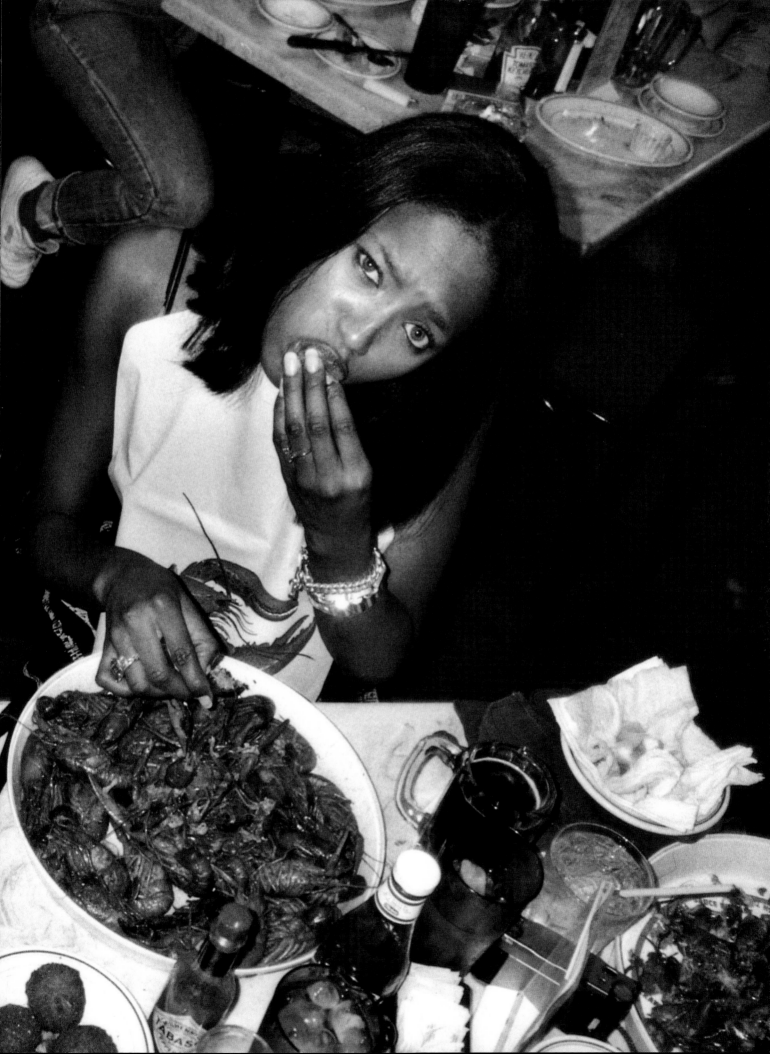

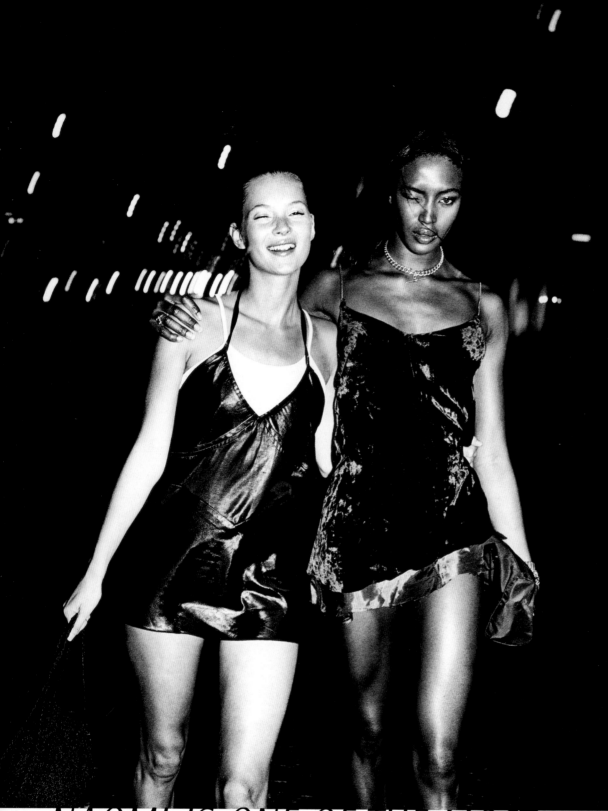

Previous spread
Photo courtesy of
Christy Turlington
New Orleans, 1994
Eating crawfish at
Amber Valletta's Wedding

This spread
Steven Klein
New York, 1994
i-D

Following spread
Peter Lindbergh
New York, 1991
Italian Vogue

NAOMI IS ONE OF THE MOST TRUTHFUL AND GENEROUS FRIENDS I HAVE EVER KNOWN. —KATE MOSS

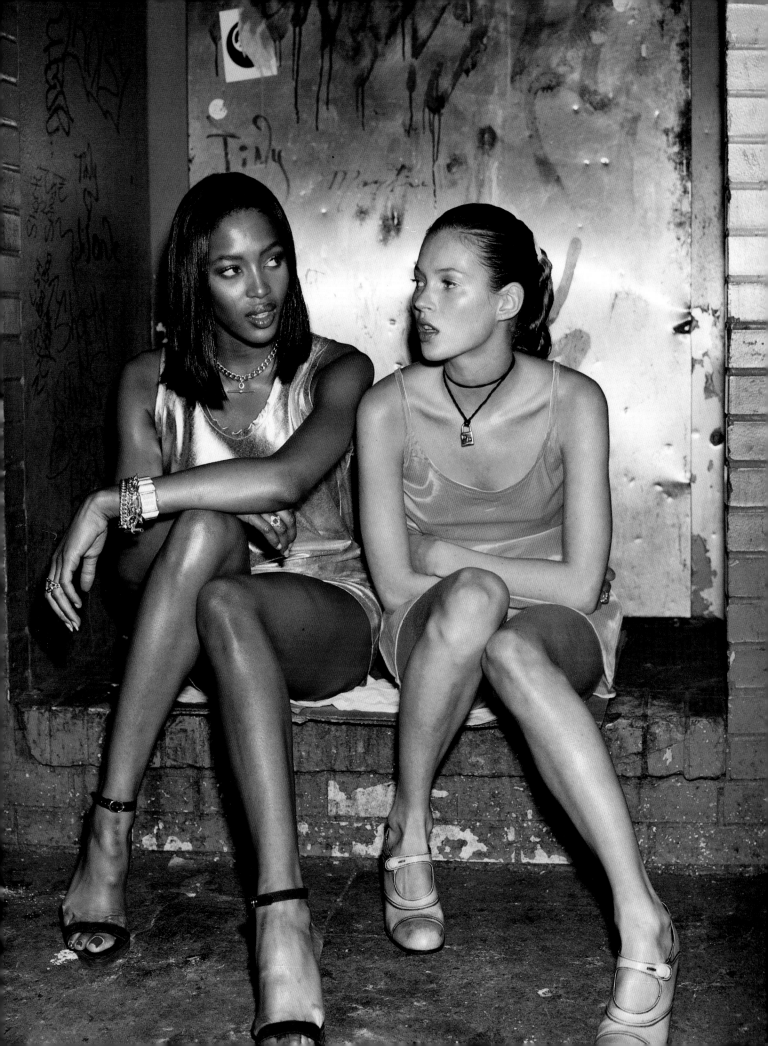

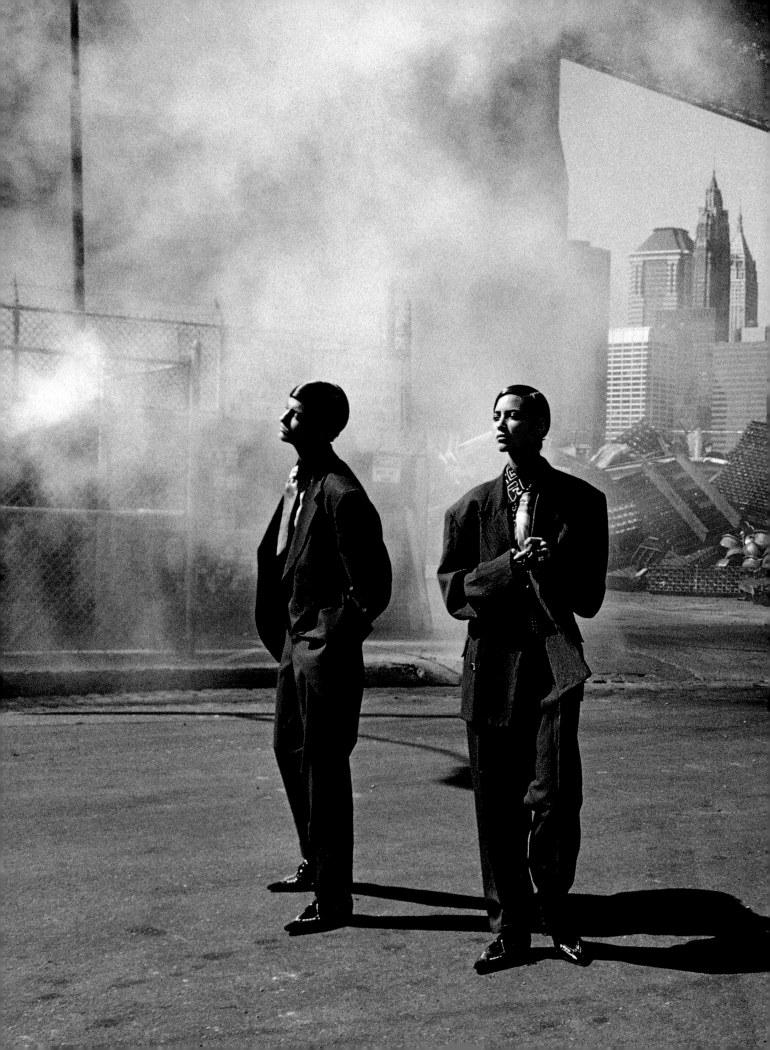

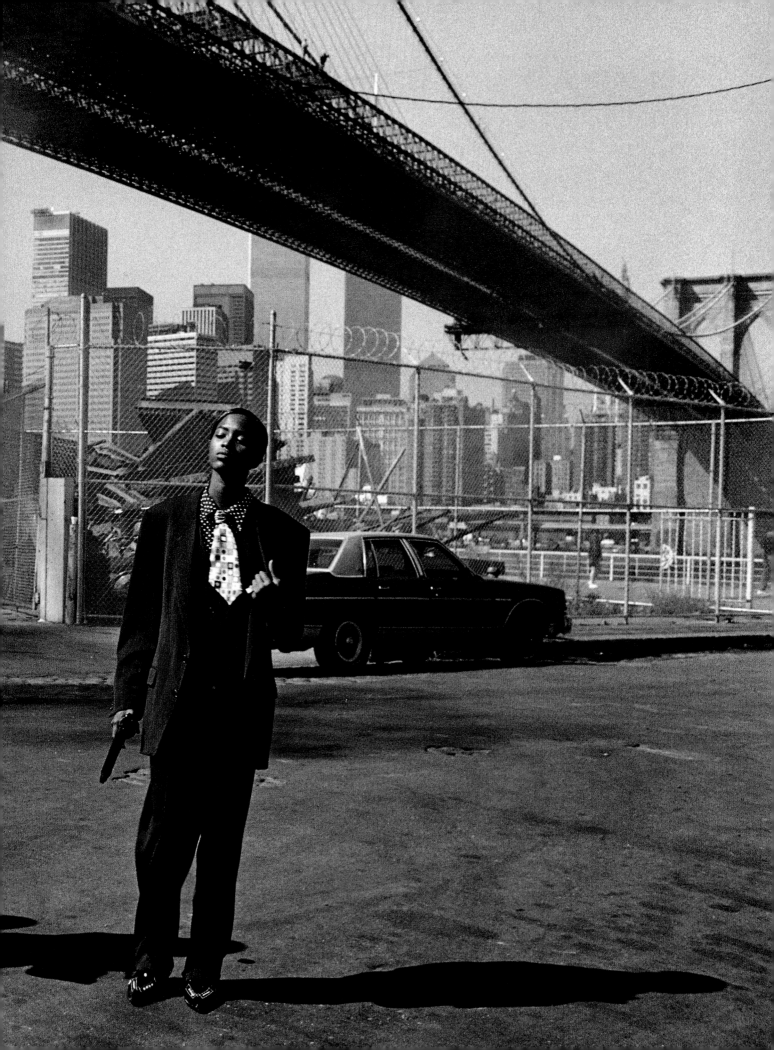

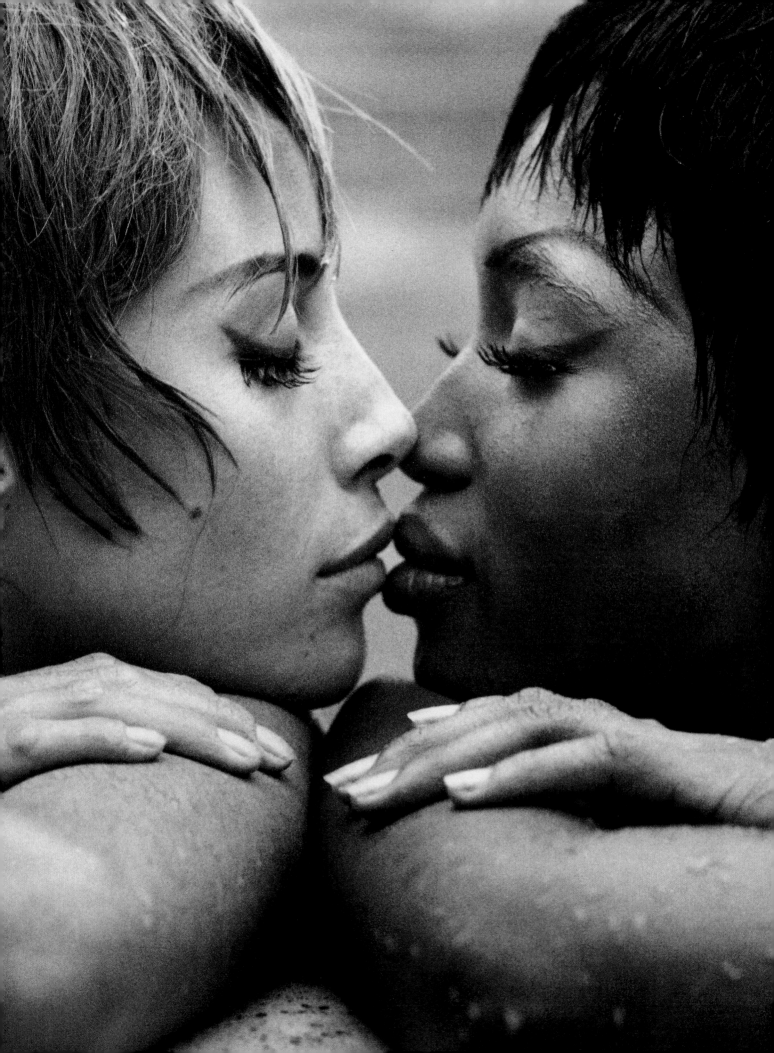

Naomi **is the** **quintessential** **free** **spirit.** **She doesn't** **really** **belong** **anywhere,** **but at the** **same** **time** **everywhere** **she goes** **is** **her home.** **She is** **eccentric** **and enigmatic.** There is

no   one quite like her in the world. I get exhausted just thinking

about keeping up with her! **—Christy Turlington**

The fashion world is, in the end, a very small one. Its stars might travel the globe, but they usually know who they'll meet at the other end.
–Naomi, from *The Face*, 1994

Steven Meisel
1989
Italian Vogue

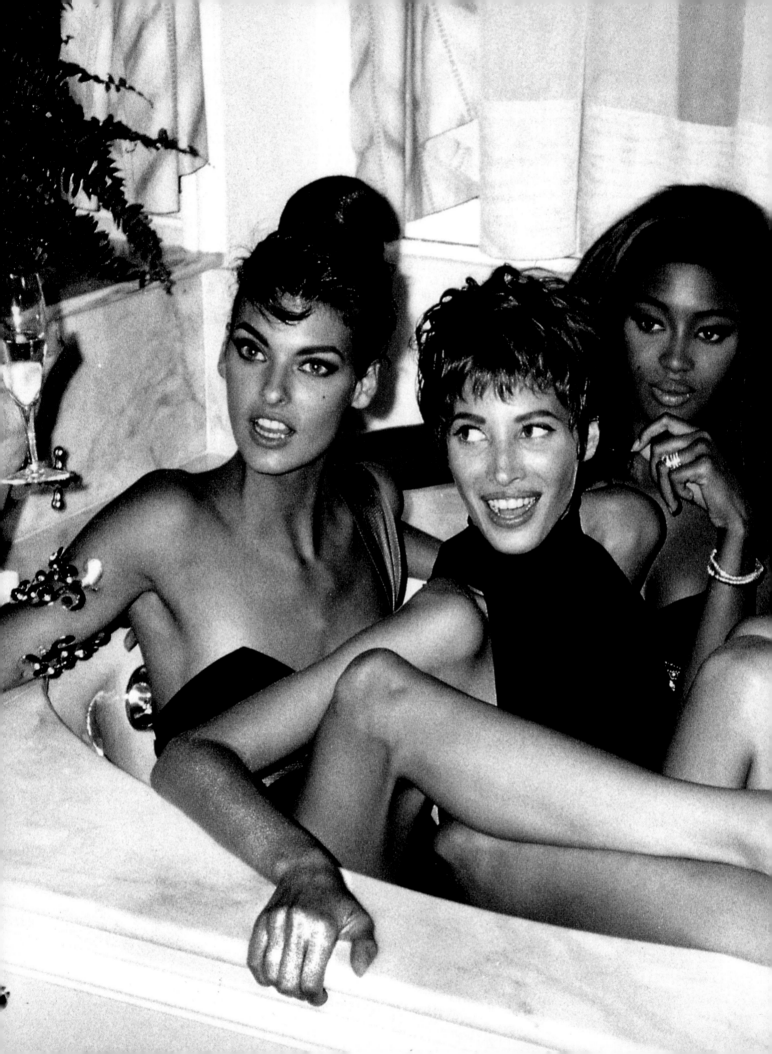

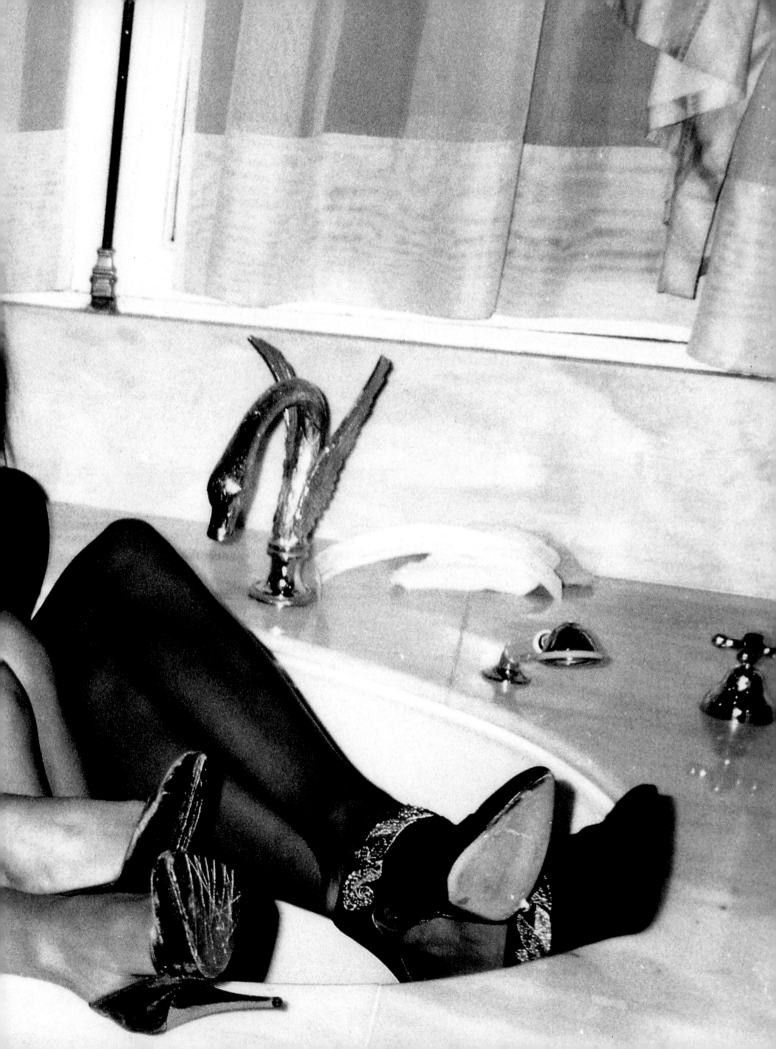

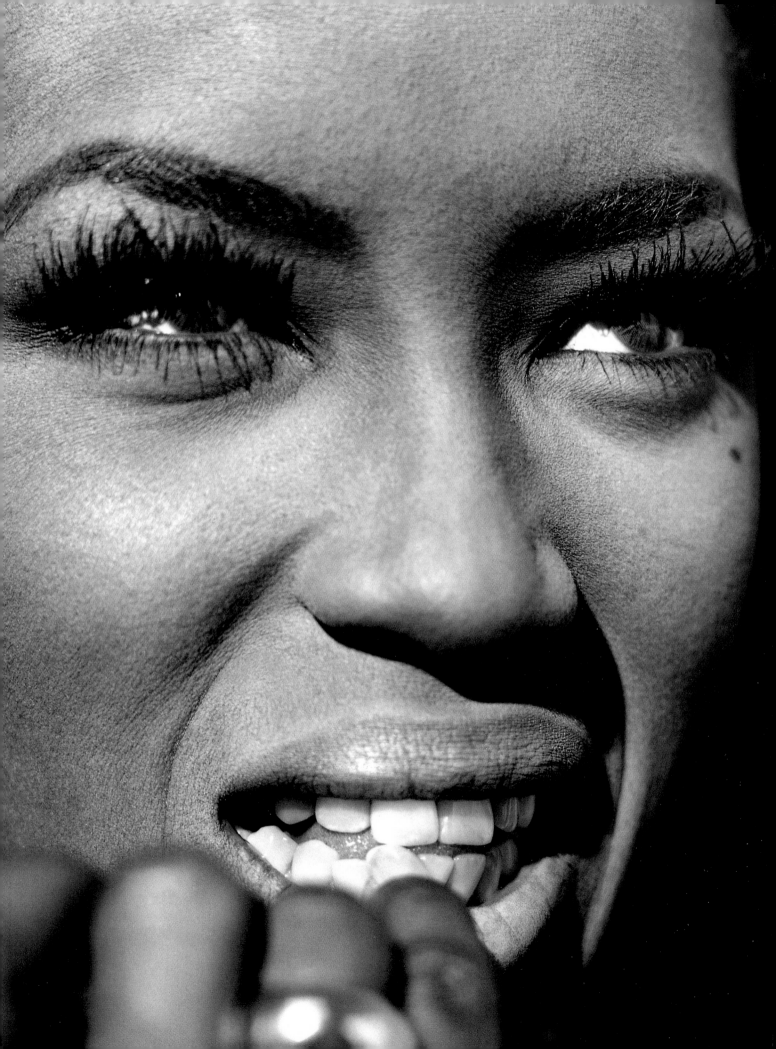

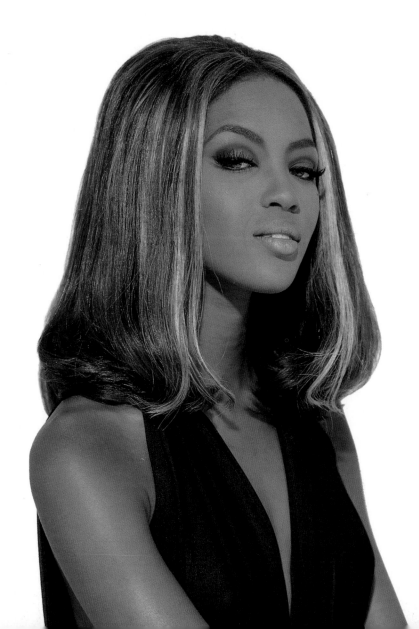

Previous spread
Roxanne Lowit
Paris, 1990
Versace couture party

This spread
Brigitte Lacombe
New York, 1991
unpublished

Following spread
Christy Turlington
1993
Naomi waiting in the Paris
airport lounge with Kate Moss

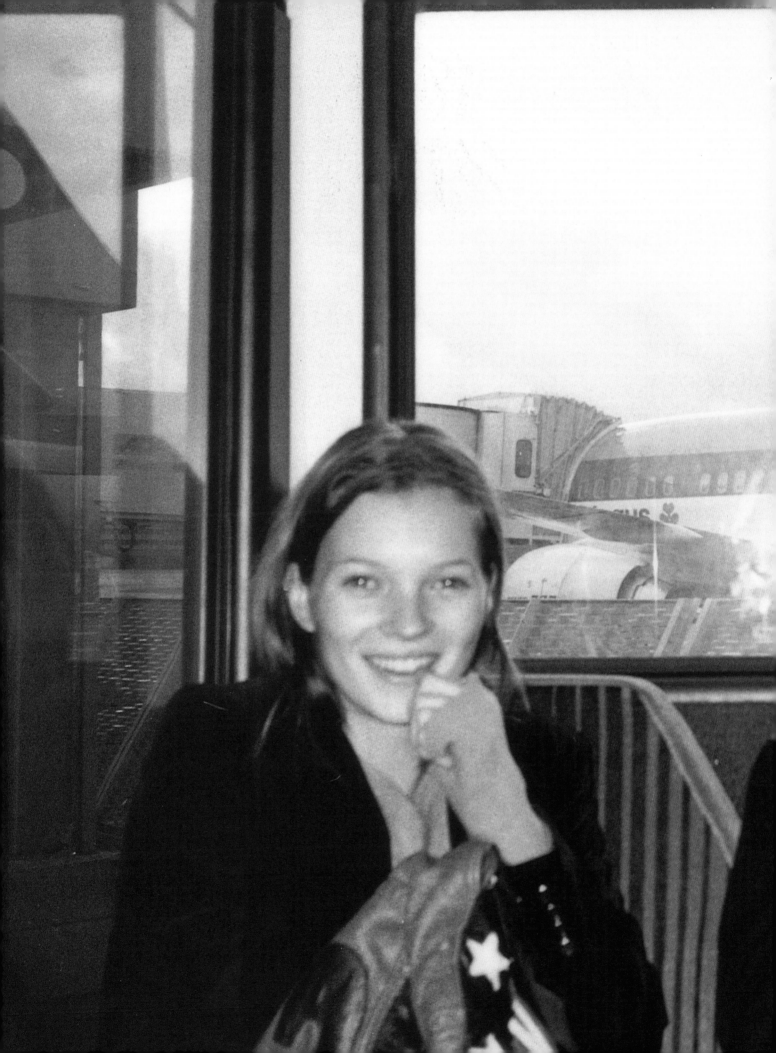

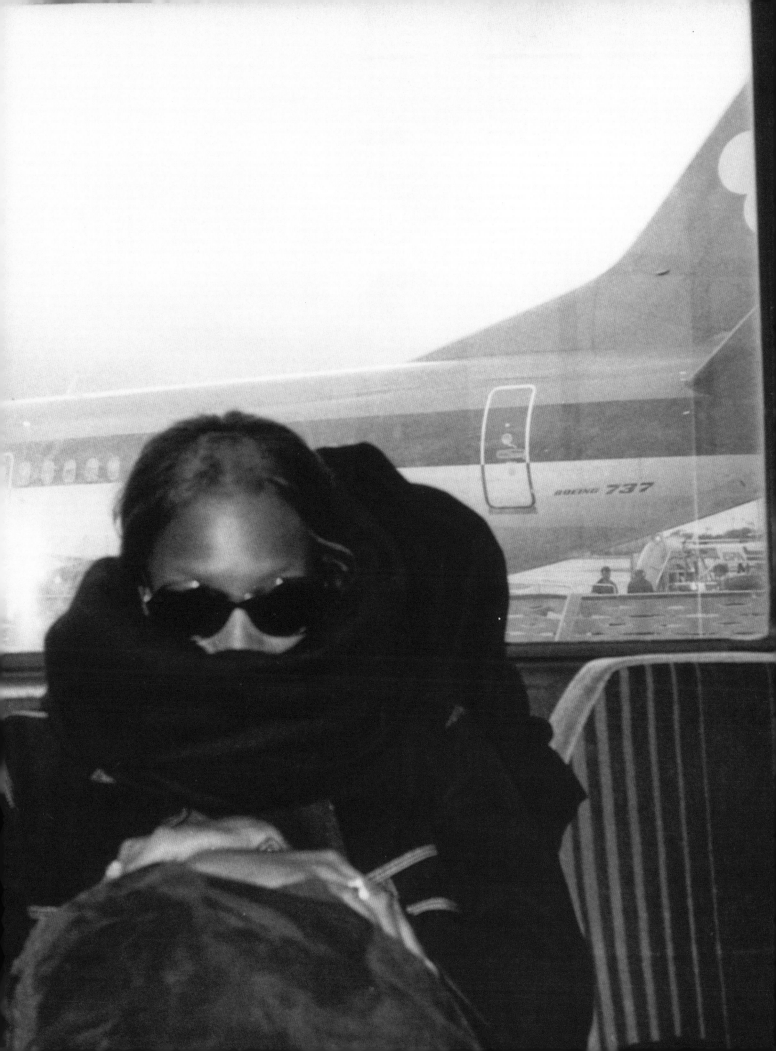

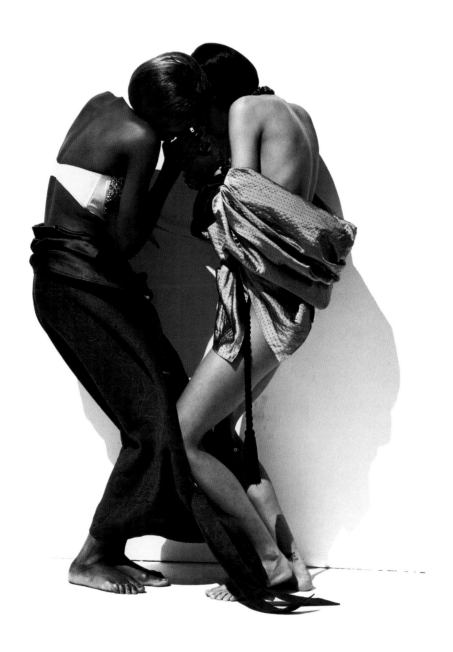

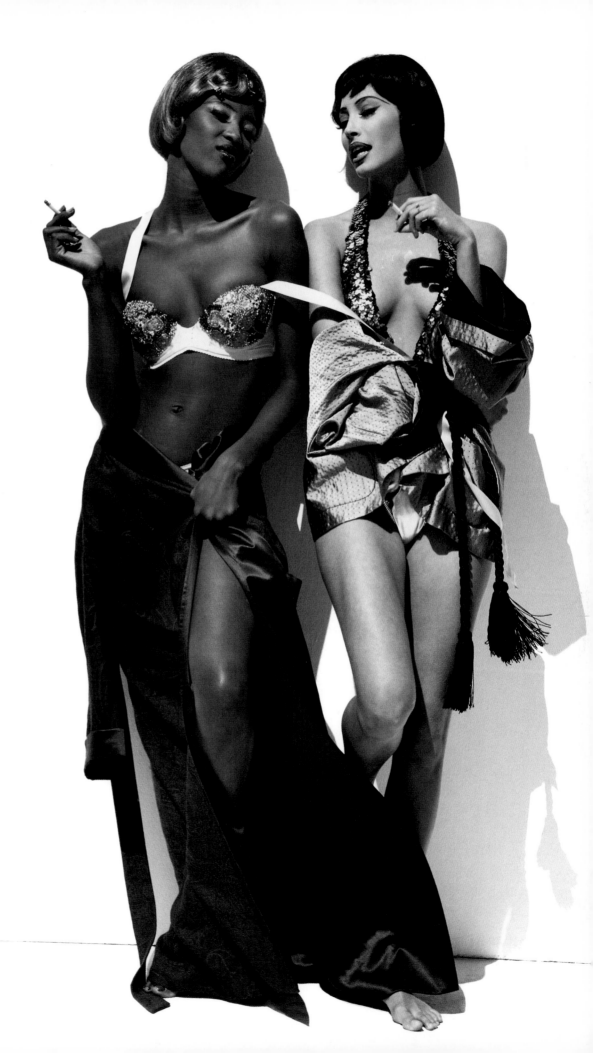

Steven Meisel
1989
Italian Vogue

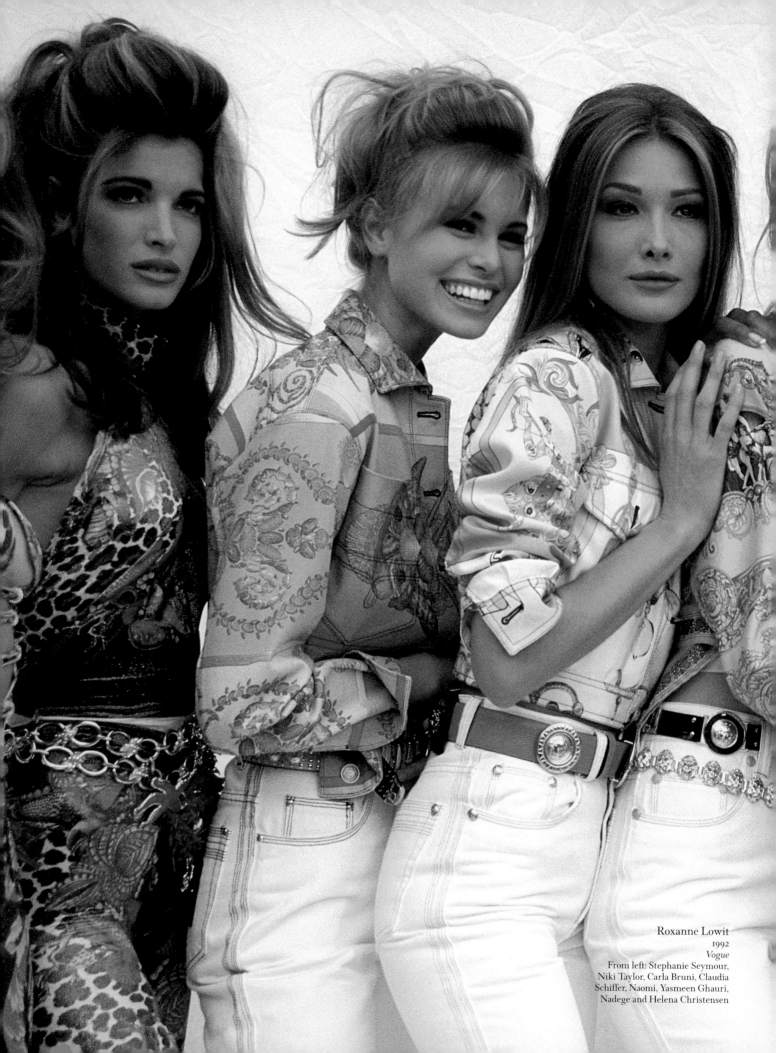

Roxanne Lowit
1992
Vogue
From left: Stephanie Seymour,
Niki Taylor, Carla Bruni, Claudia
Schiffer, Naomi, Yasmeen Ghauri,
Nadege and Helena Christensen

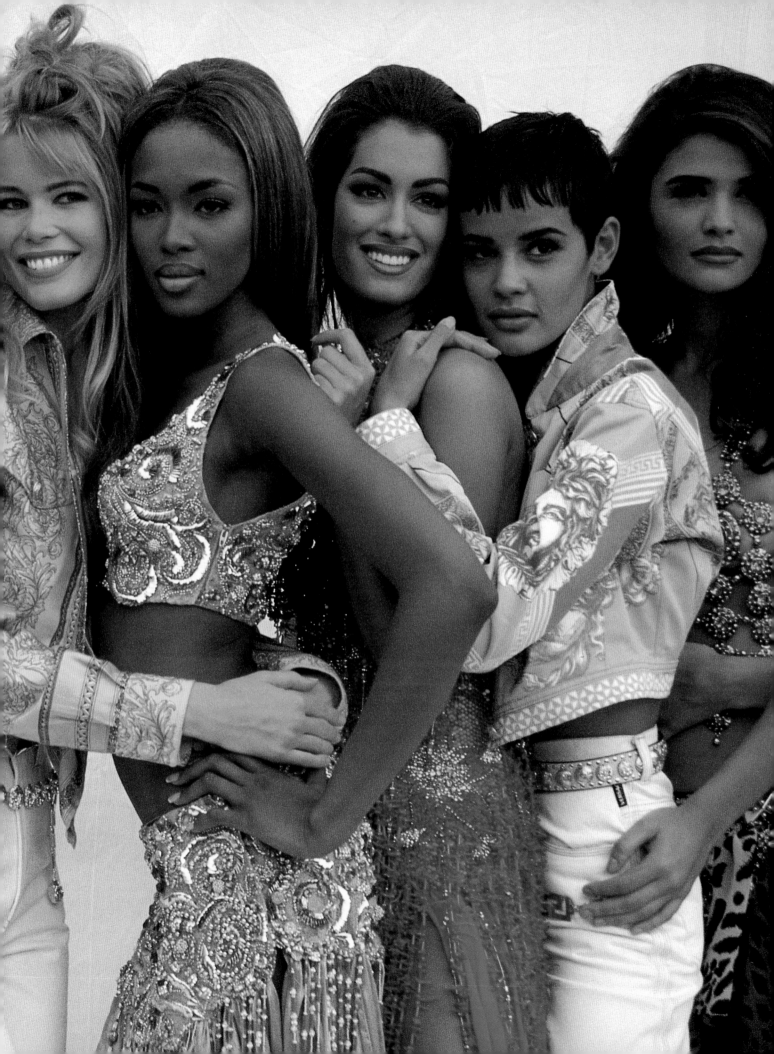

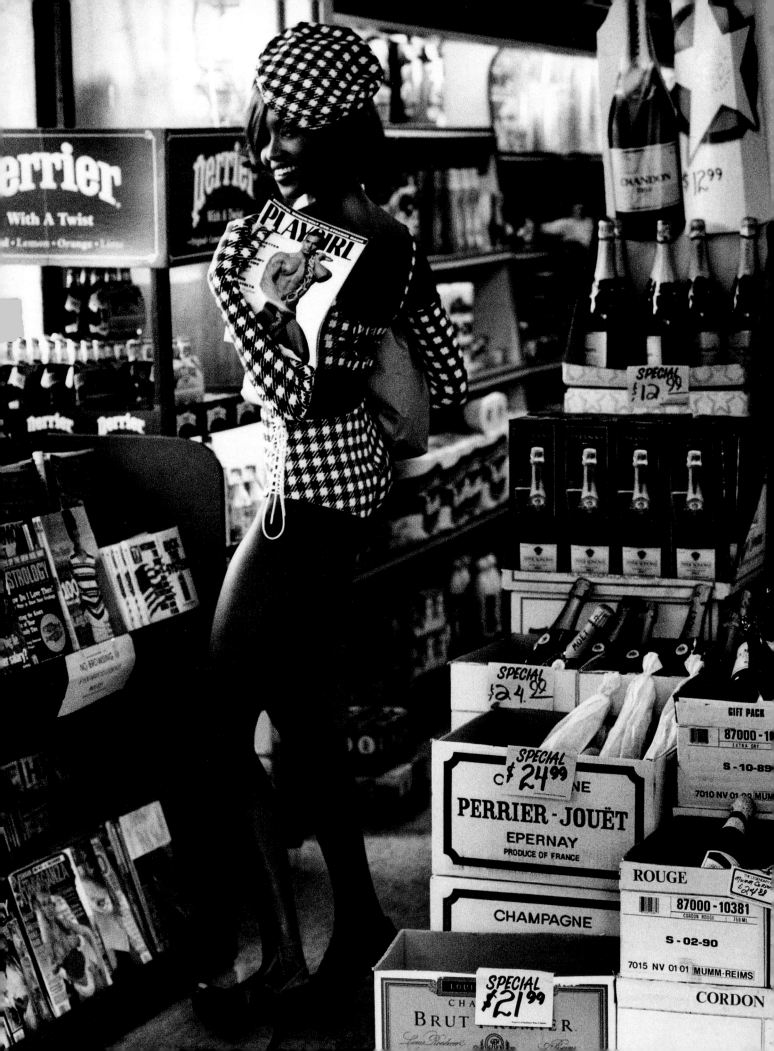

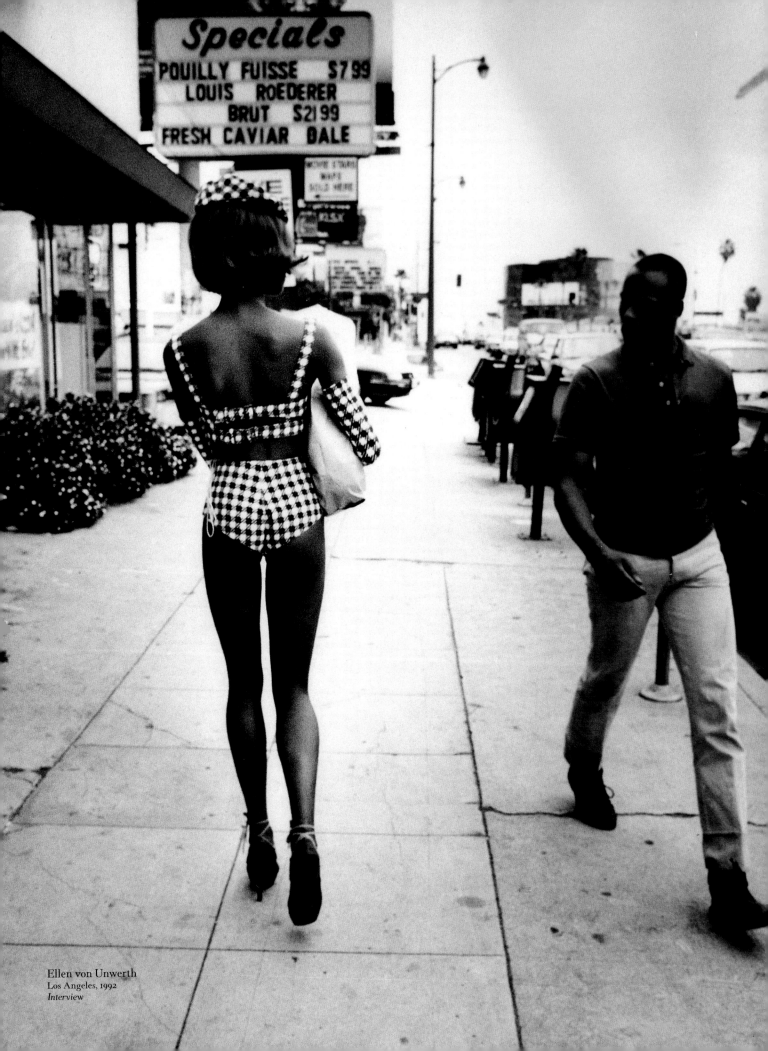

Ellen von Unwerth
Los Angeles, 1992
Interview

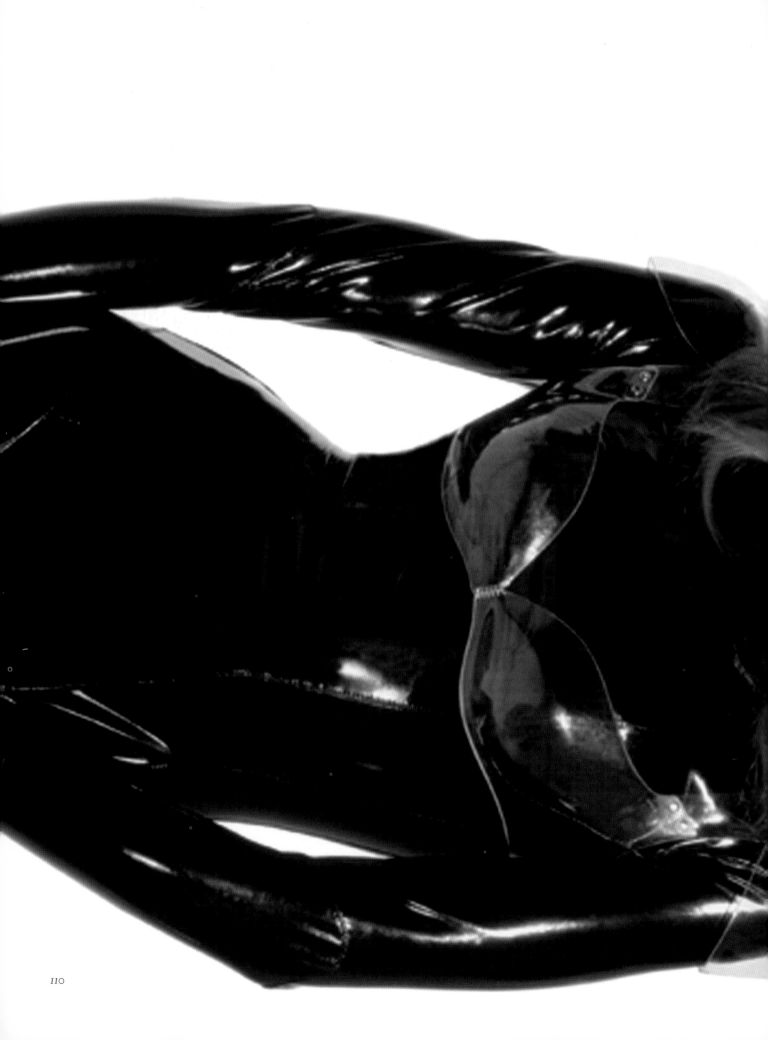

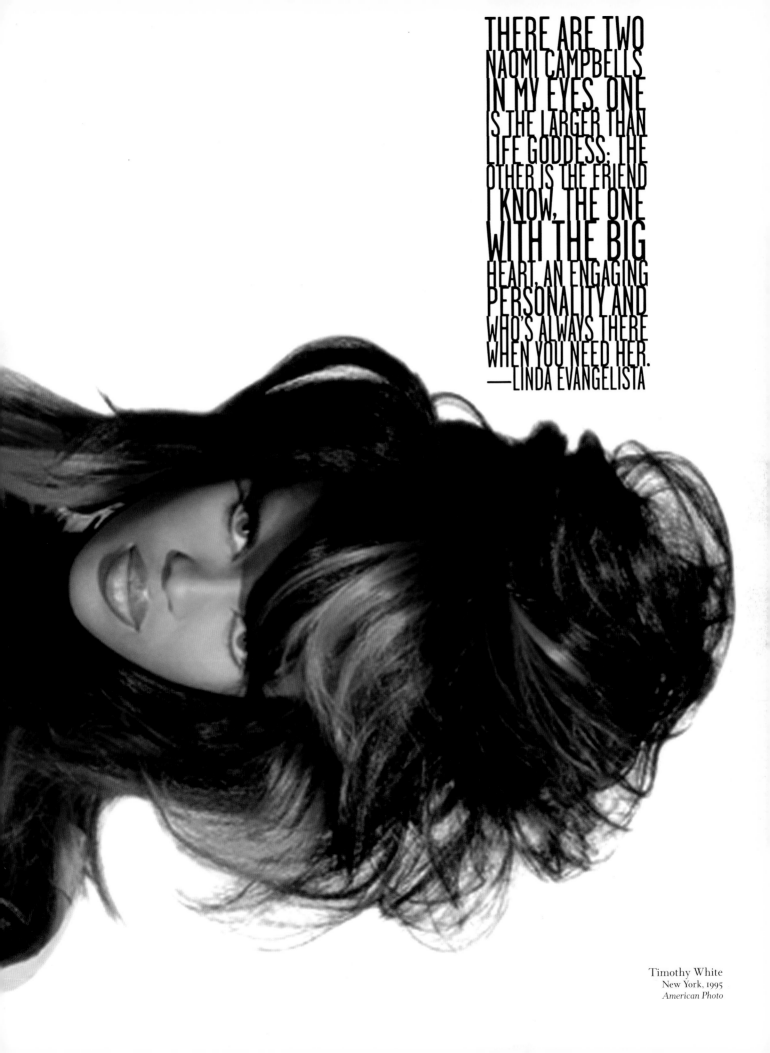

THERE ARE TWO
NAOMI CAMPBELLS
IN MY EYES. ONE
IS THE LARGER THAN
LIFE GODDESS; THE
OTHER IS THE FRIEND
I KNOW, THE ONE
WITH THE BIG
HEART, AN ENGAGING
PERSONALITY, AND
WHO'S ALWAYS THERE
WHEN YOU NEED HER.
—LINDA EVANGELISTA

Timothy White
New York, 1995
American Photo

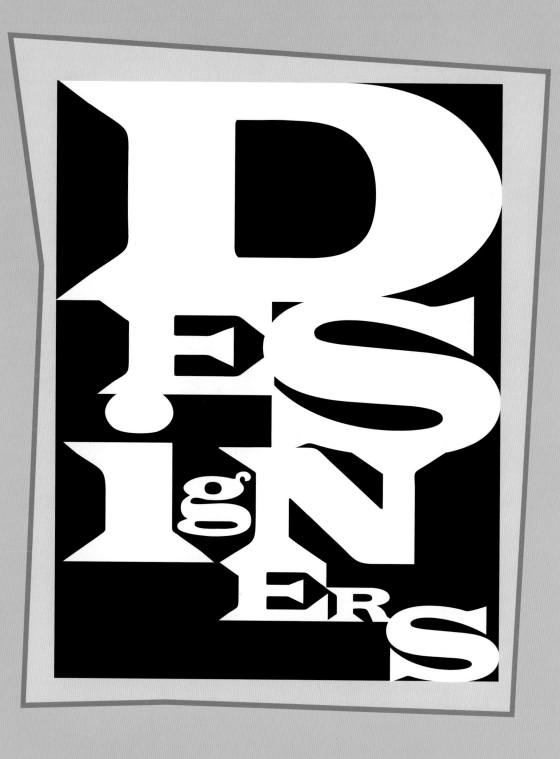

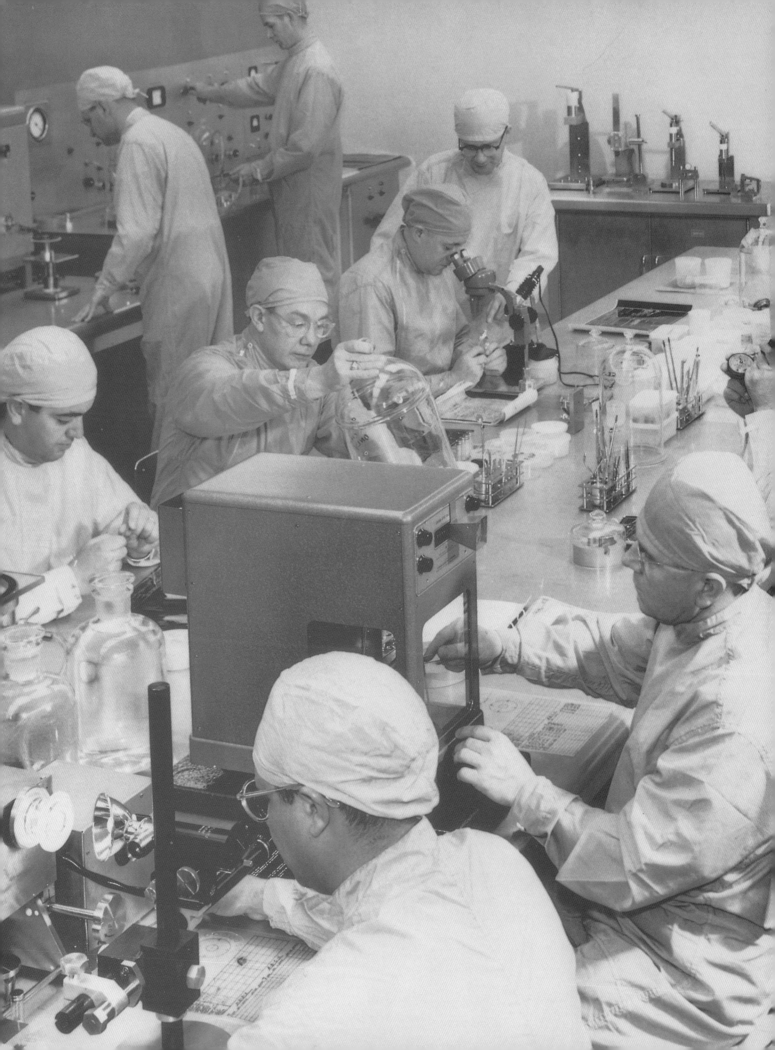

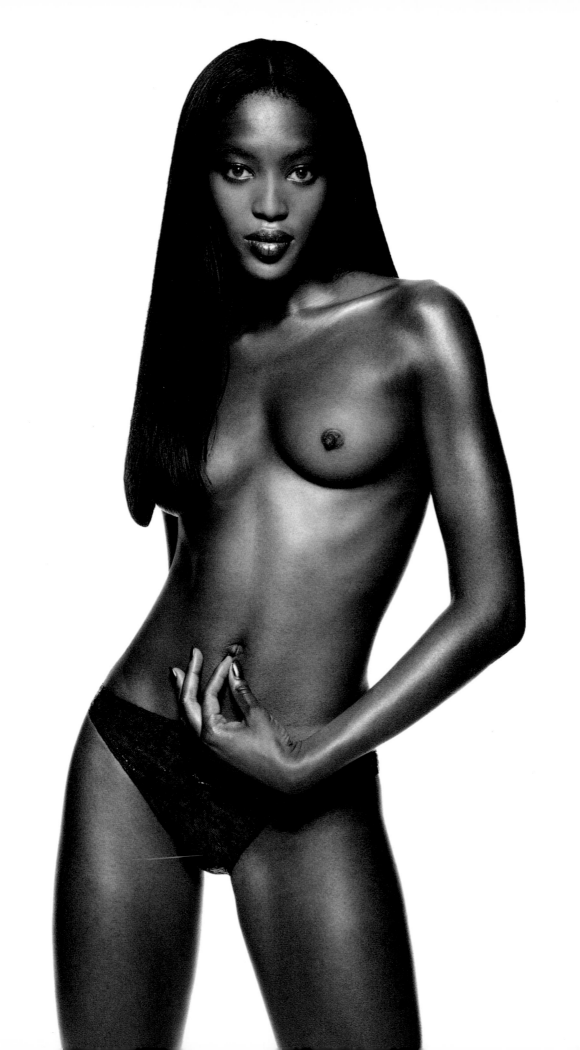

"Fashion spreads are about ideas, inspired by a mood.

Personally, I wear whatever I want to. But some people

open a magazine and think, 'God, I've got to look like that.'

That's when it's like, wait a minute. You look at it

to get ideas, not to starve yourself and get anorexic."

–Naomi, from *The Face*, 1994

Thierry Le Gouès
1994
unpublished

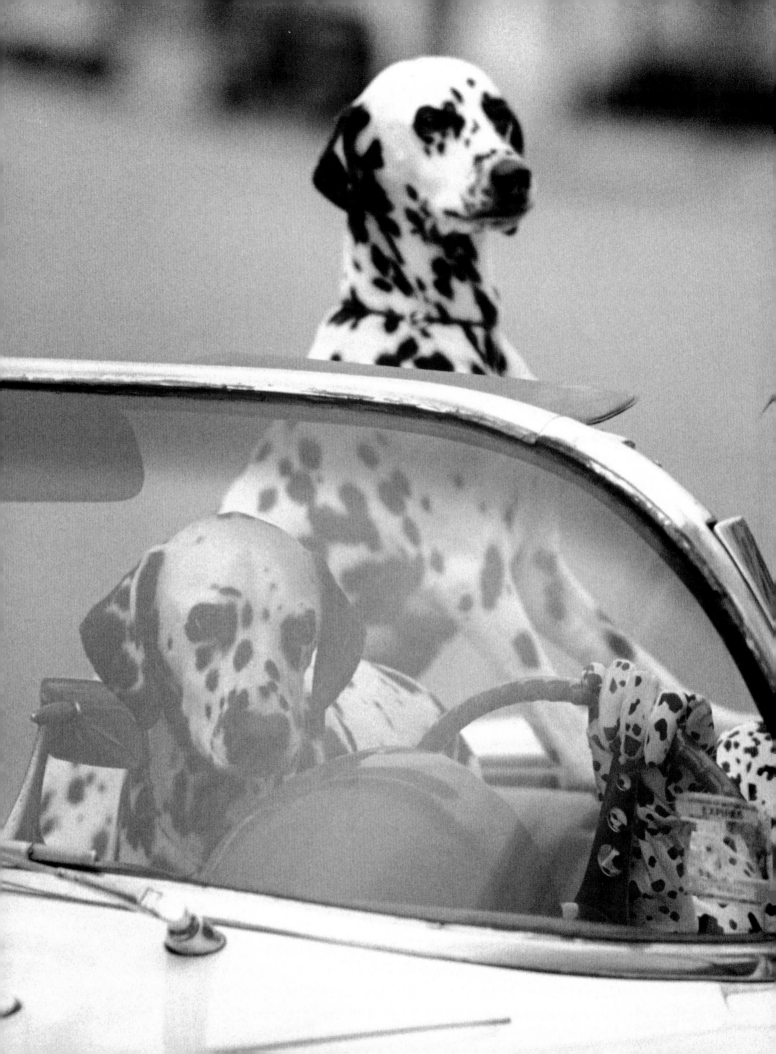

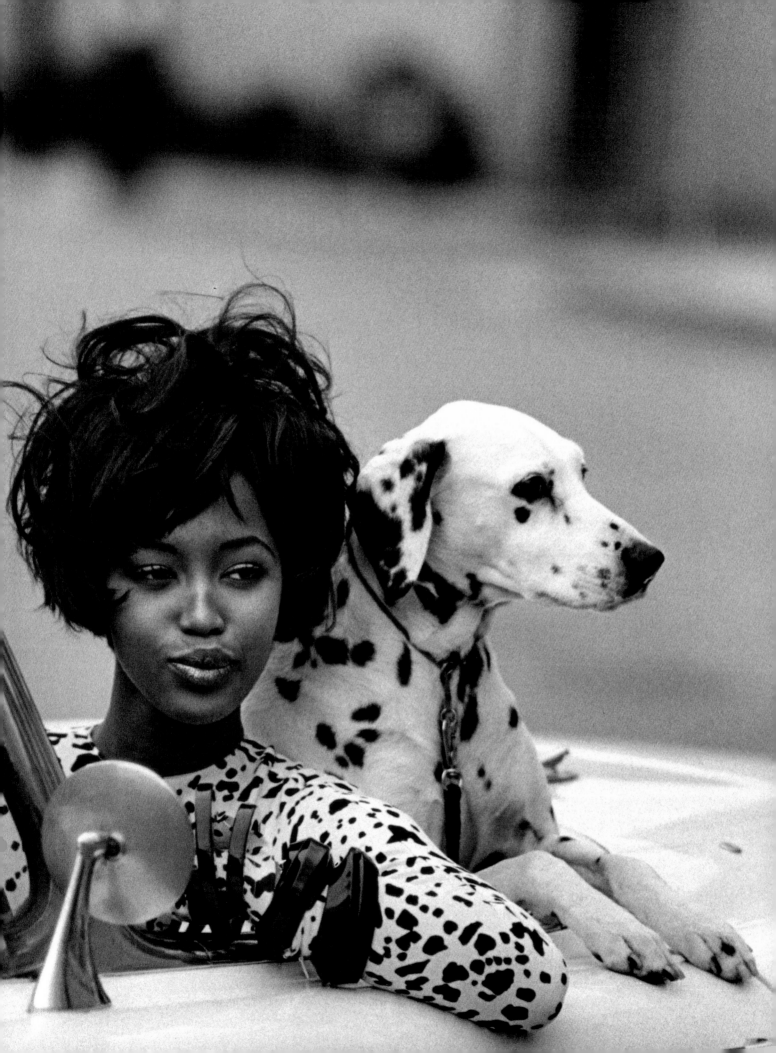

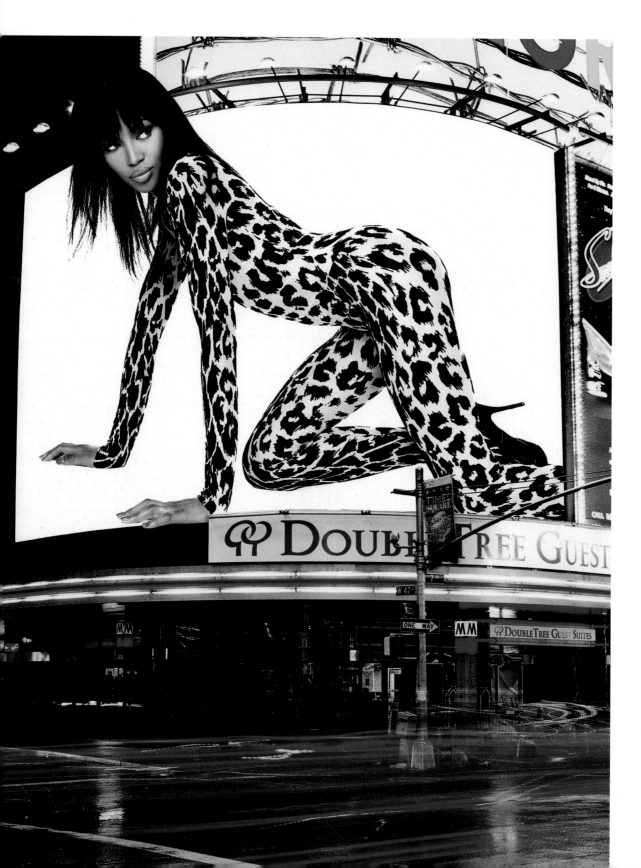

Previous spread
Peter Lindbergh
1990
Vogue

This page
Thierry Le Gouès
1995
Allure

Opposite
Sante D'Orazio
New York, 1992
British Vogue

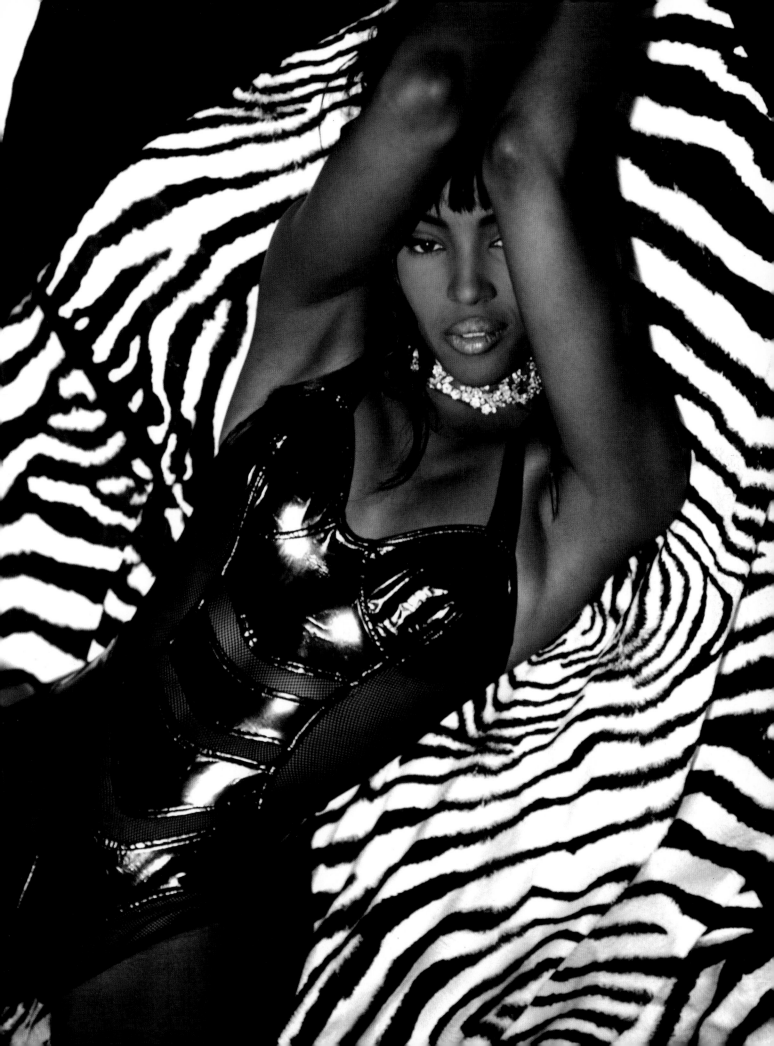

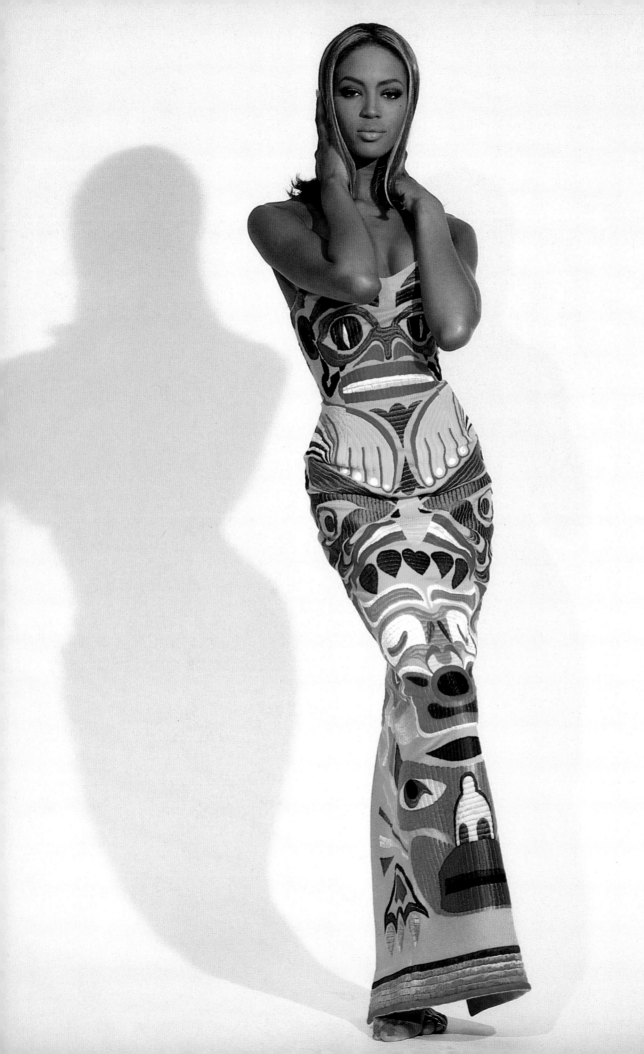

Not
only do
people
of all
kinds gravitate
to Naomi—the
landscape
gravitates
to her, trees
gravitate to
her—when she
walks into a
room, it
becomes
much
smaller
for her
grand
presence.
—Isaac Mizrahi

Brigitte Lacombe
New York, 1991
Time Magazine

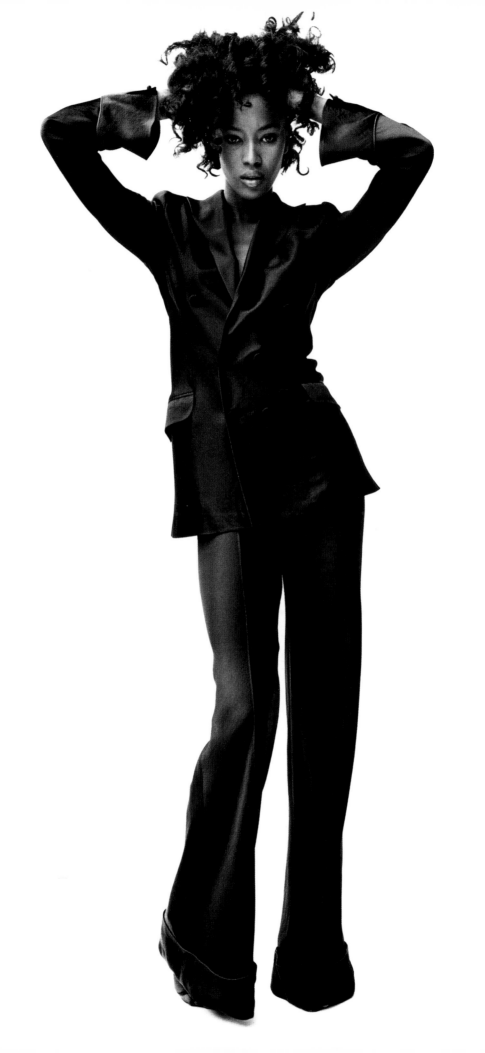

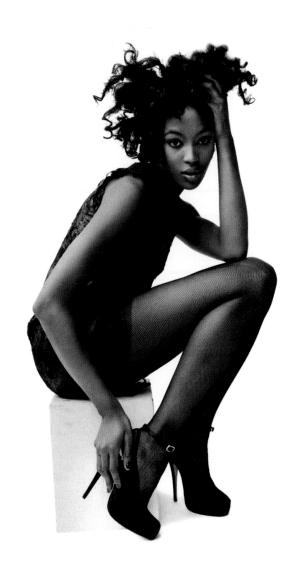

Mario Testino
Paris, 1994
Allure

Following spread
Mario Testino
Paris, 1996
Versace campaign

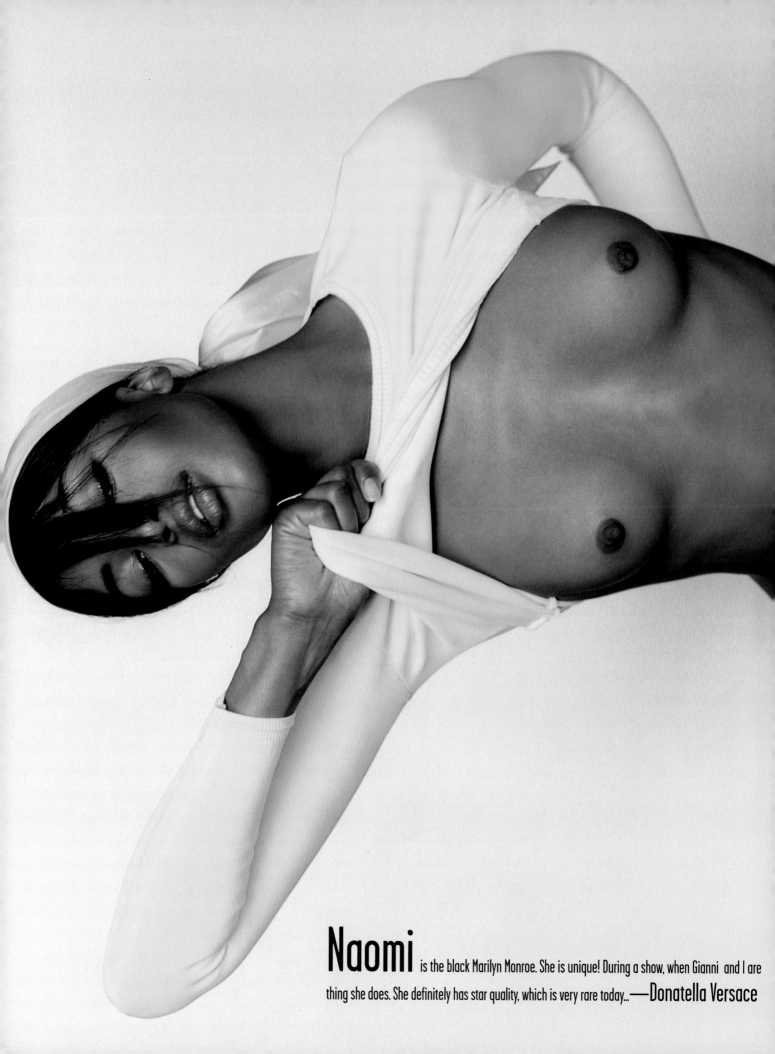

Naomi is the black Marilyn Monroe. She is unique! During a show, when Gianni and I are thing she does. She definitely has star quality, which is very rare today...—**Donatella Versace**

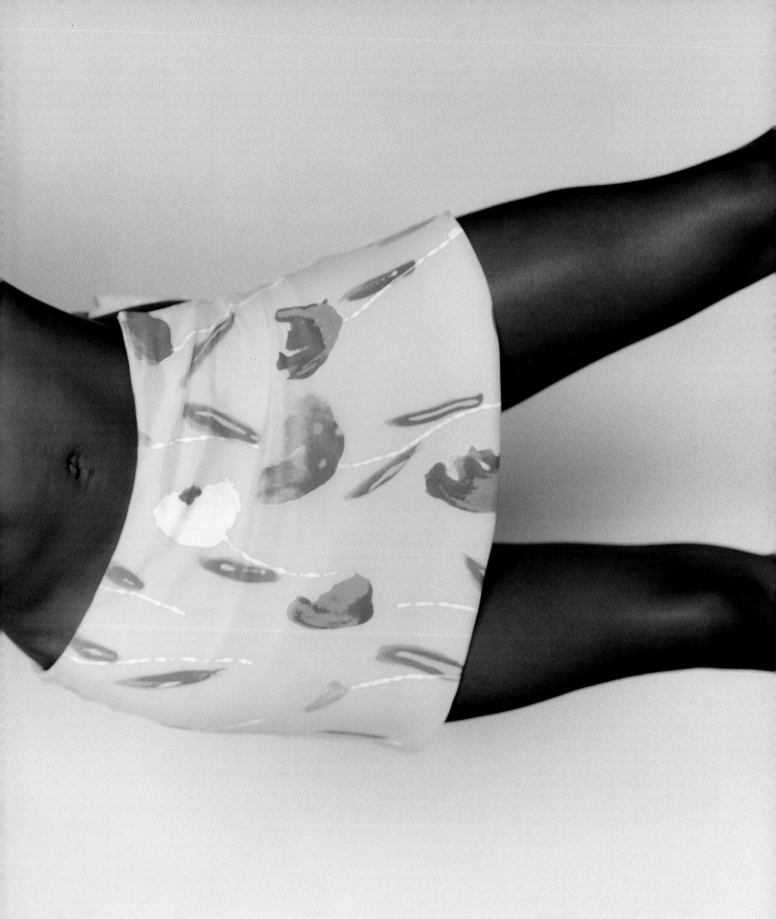

watching together, he will say, "The outfit is good, but the fact that Naomi is modeling it makes the outfit absolutely fantastic!" Naomi gives great emotion to every-

"Black girls from south London aren't meant to make it quite this big." –Naomi, from *Attitude*, 1994

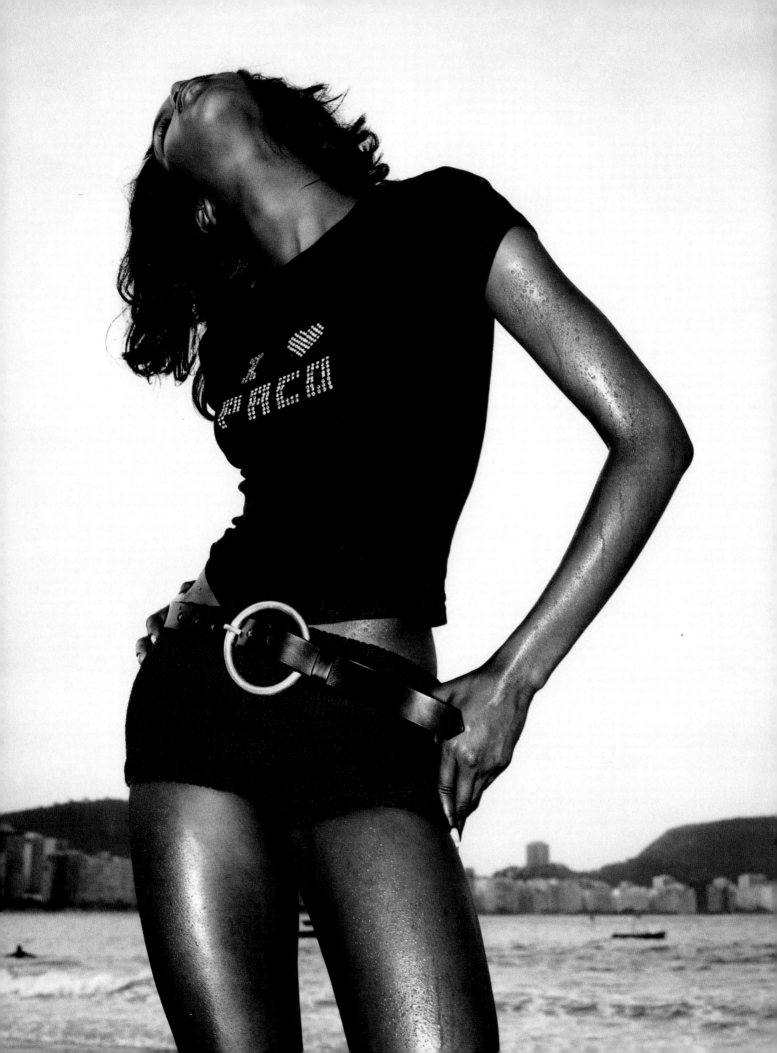

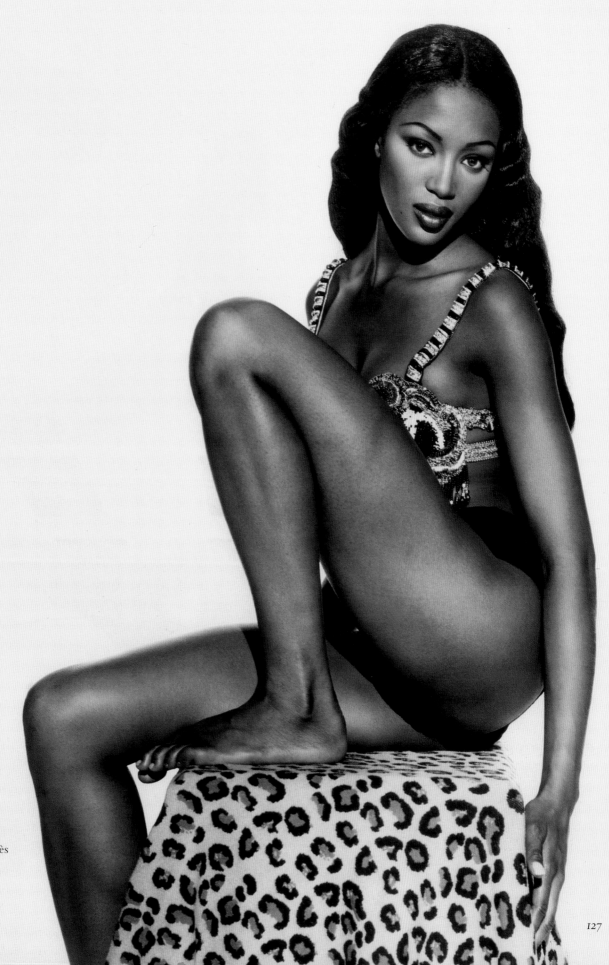

Thierry Le Gouès
1992
Vogue Homme

Opposite
Mario Testino
Rio de Janiero, 1994
French Glamour

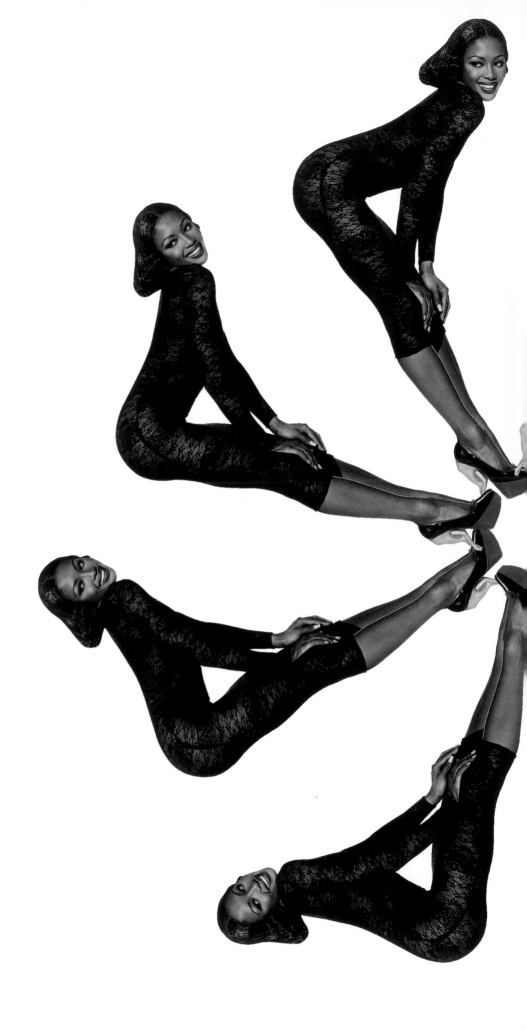

Thierry Le Goués
1992
Vogue Homme

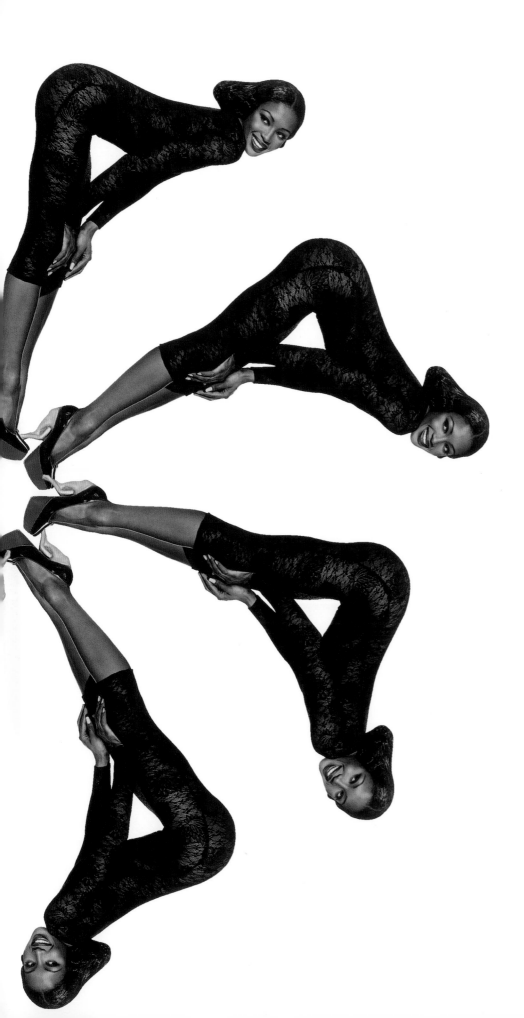

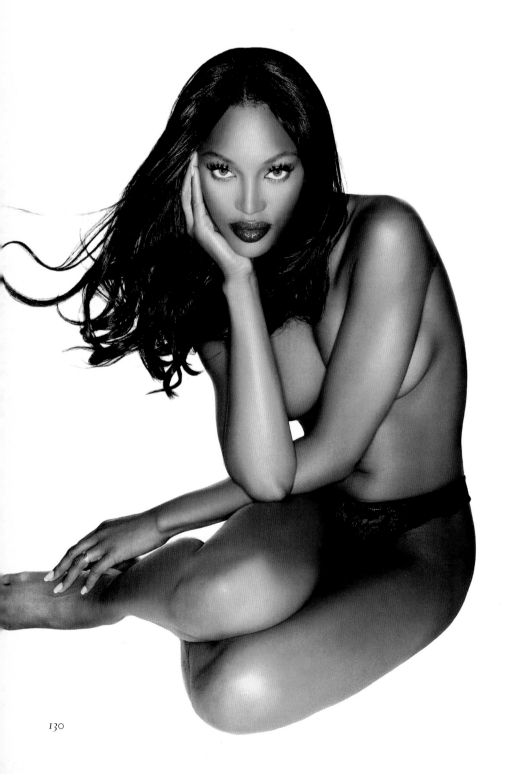

Michael Thompson
New York, 1995
British Esquire

Opposite
Matthew Rolston
New York, 1994
Spanish Vogue

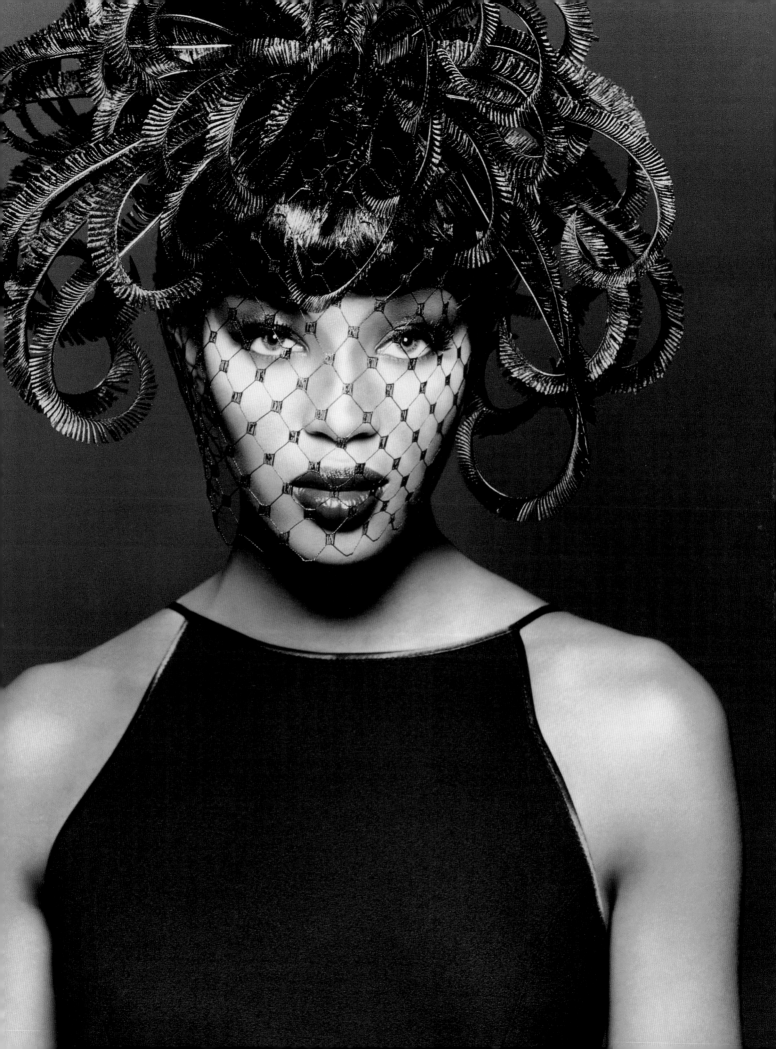

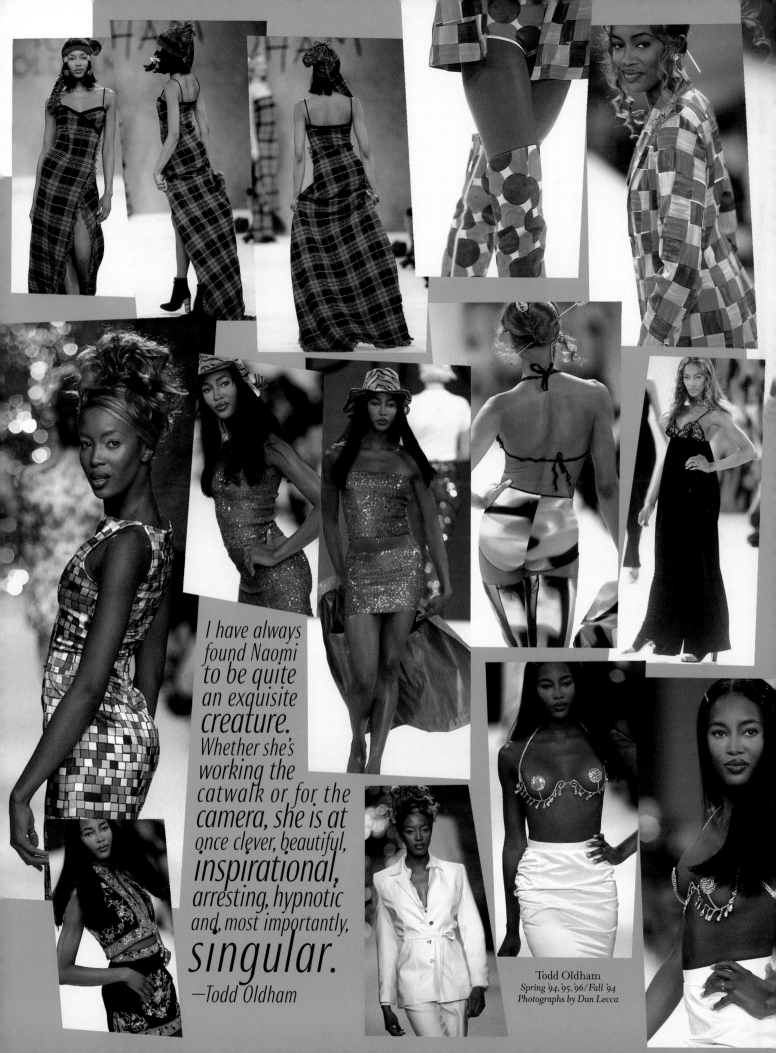

I have always found Naomi to be quite an exquisite *creature.* Whether she's working the catwalk or for the camera, she is at once clever, beautiful, **inspirational,** arresting, hypnotic and, most importantly, **singular.**
—Todd Oldham

Todd Oldham
Spring '94, '95, '96/Fall '94
Photographs by Dan Lecca

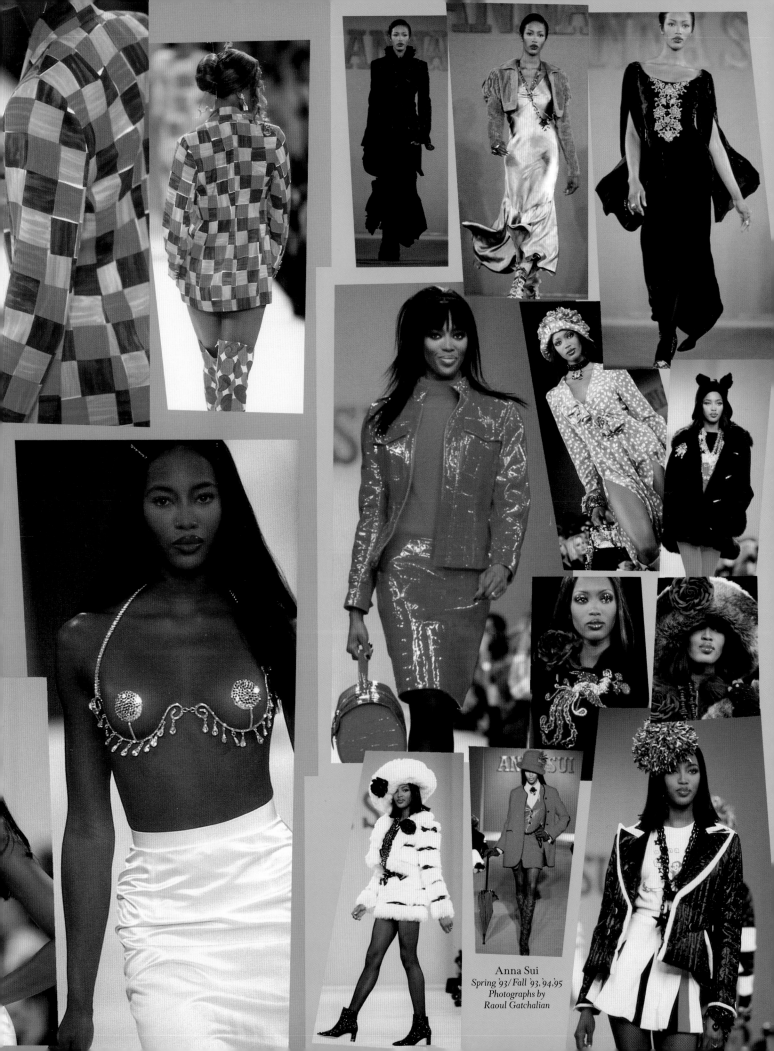

Anna Sui
Spring '93/ Fall '93, '94, '95
Photographs by
Raoul Gatchalian

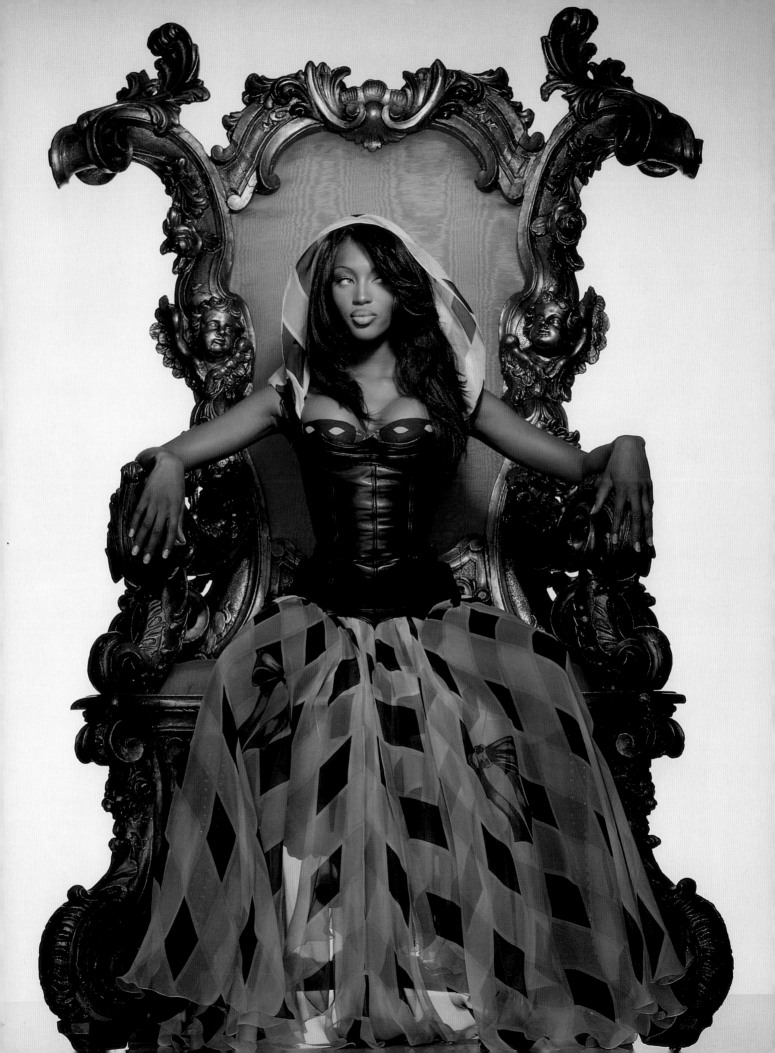

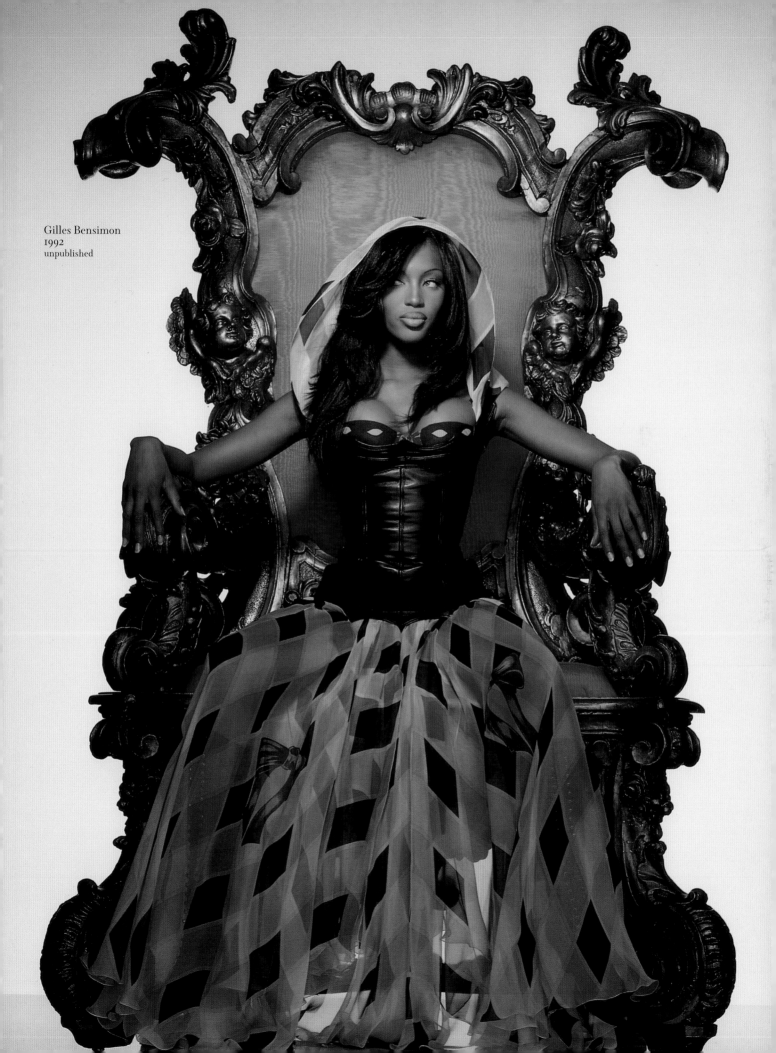

Gilles Bensimon
1992
unpublished

*E*very season my inspiration

of sources as diverse as Worth to David Lean.

*H*owever, when it comes

*N*aomi's dress every season, she is the

only inspiration I need.

"I don't always wear underwear. When I'm in the heat especially, I can't wear it. Like, if I'm wearing a flowing dress, why do I have to wear underwear?"
—Naomi, from *Arthur Elgort's Models Manual*

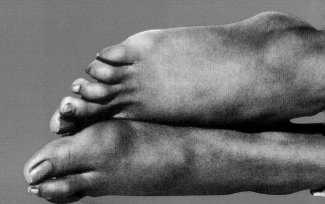

Gilles Bensimon
1992
French Elle

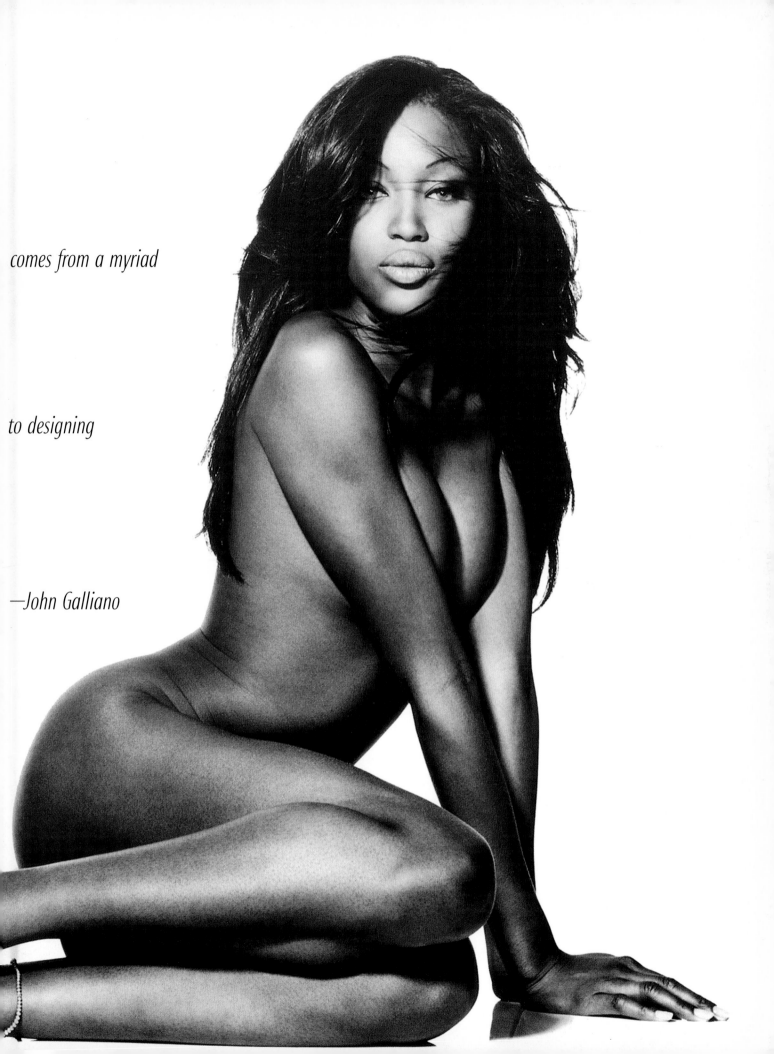

comes from a myriad

to designing

—John Galliano

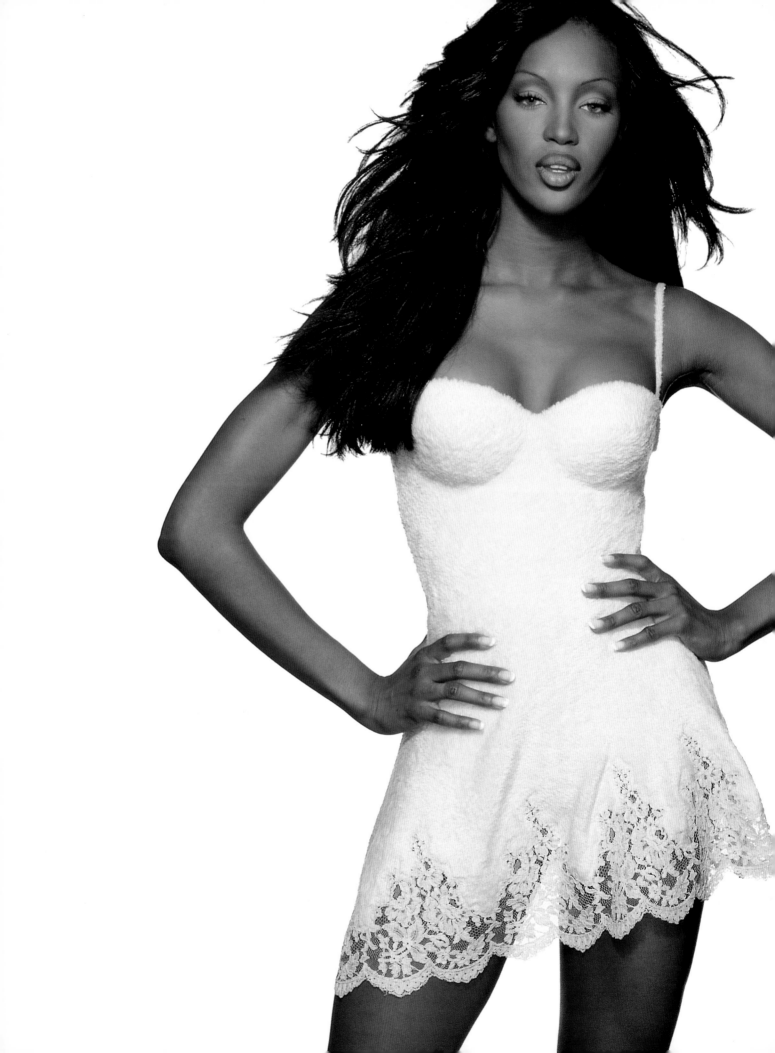

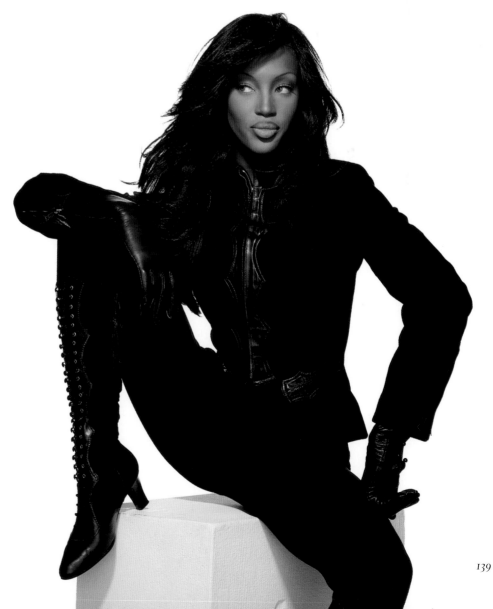

Gilles Bensimon
1992
Elle

Acknowledgments

This book is dedicated to my family and friends, and is in memory of Johnny Chappoulis.

First and foremost, a huge thanks to my colleagues Carole White, Chris Owen, and Carlton Gardner for their professional support, generosity, and friendship.

Many, many thanks to: Valerie Morris, Pierre Blackwood, Lisa Smith and Stephanie Pierre at Elite Premier, Didier Fernandez, Raphael Santin and Sabine Killinger at Elite Paris, David Brown at Riccardo Gay, Stuart Cameron, Paul Rowland, and Jennifer Ramey at Women Model Management, Allan Grubman and Mark Steverson at Grubman Indursky, Quincy Jones and Hayden, Iman, Bethann Hardison, Azzedine Alaïa, John Galliano, Gianni and Donatella Versace, Gianni Nunnari, Candy Price, B-B, Danielle Locks, Sara Foley and Paul Cavacco at *Harper's Bazaar*, Andre Leon Talley, Jung Richard, Jim Johnson, Janet Johnson, François Nars, Jennie Lister-Oldfield, Orlando Pita, Christy Turlington, Kate Moss, Linda Evangelista, Lisa Smith, Isaac Mizrahi, Todd Oldham, Elton John, Patti LaBelle, Bono, and Eric Clapton. Special thanks to Bruce Ramsay, Sandy Gilbert, and Charles Miers.

Major thanks to all of the photographers and contributors without whom this book could not have been made.

The Publisher would like to thank Gabon Designers Africa and Consty Eka of Cekam Productions for conducting the interview appearing in this book.

Photographers featured

Richard Avedon
Gilles Bensimon
Anton Corbijn
Patrick Demarchelier
Sante D'Orazio
Steven Klein
Herbie Knott
Brigitte Lacombe
Thierry Le Gouès
Mark Liddell
Peter Lindbergh
Roxanne Lowit
Steven Meisel
Jack Pierson
Huggy Ragnarsson
Herb Ritts
Matthew Rolston
Paolo Roversi
Mario Testino
Michael Thompson
Ellen von Unwerth
Albert Watson
Timothy White
Michael Williams

Section opener credits

Photographers: Corbis-Bettmann
Musicians: The Bettmann Archive
Models: The Bettmann Archive
Designers: Corbis-Bettmann
(opposite: Bettmann Newsphotos)

Interview section, photograph taken from *Swan*, Naomi Campbell, author/Caroline Upcher, writer; published by William Heinemann Ltd. (an imprint of Reed International Books, Ltd., 1994)

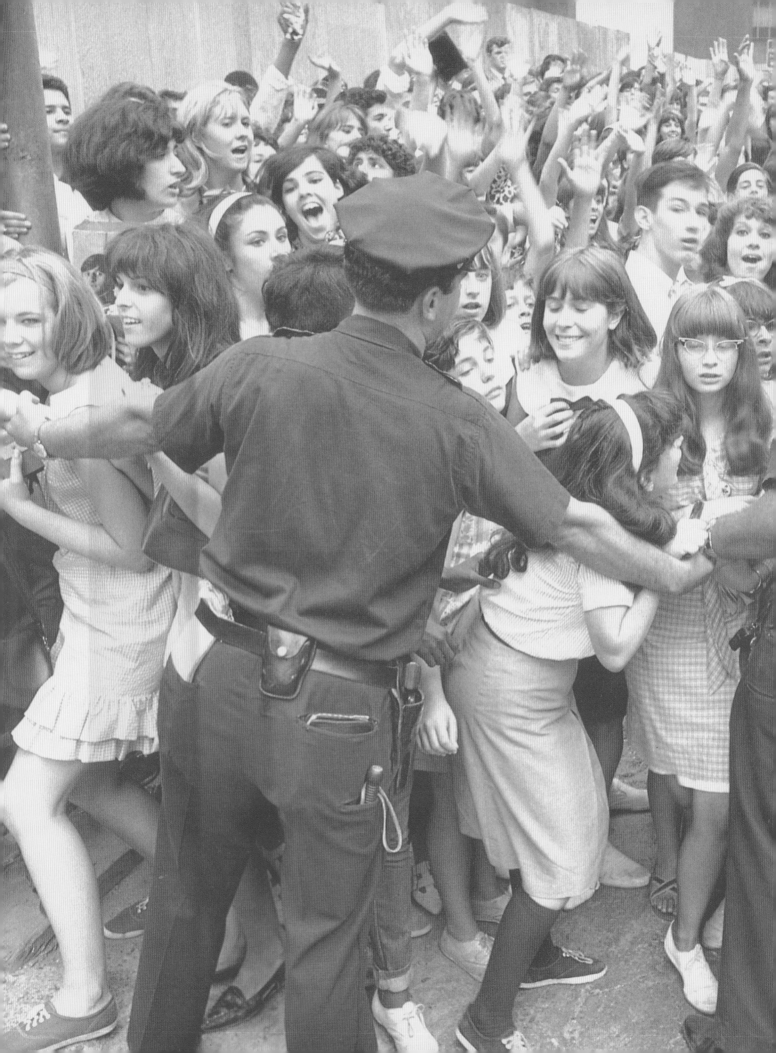

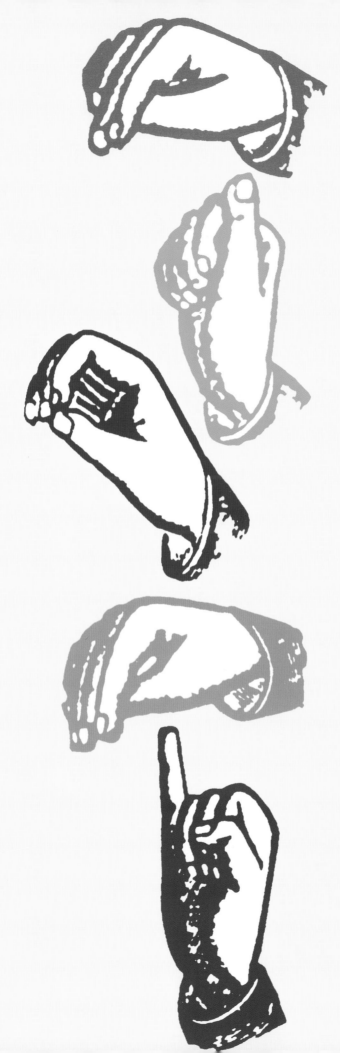

Timothy White
New York, 1995
Esquire

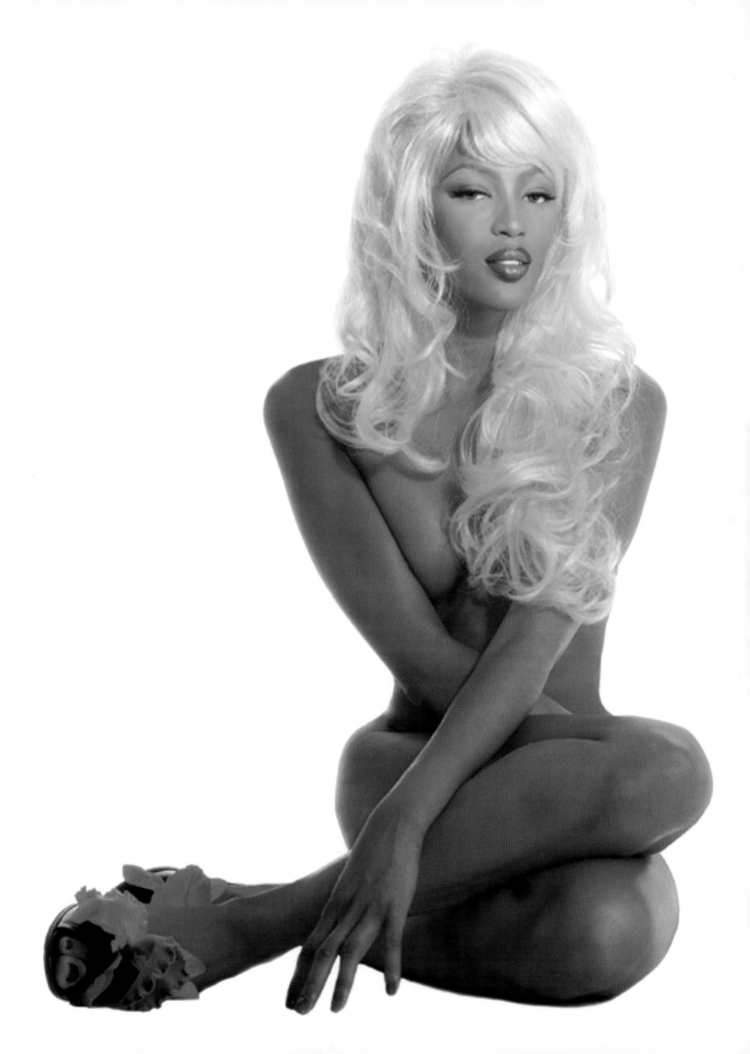

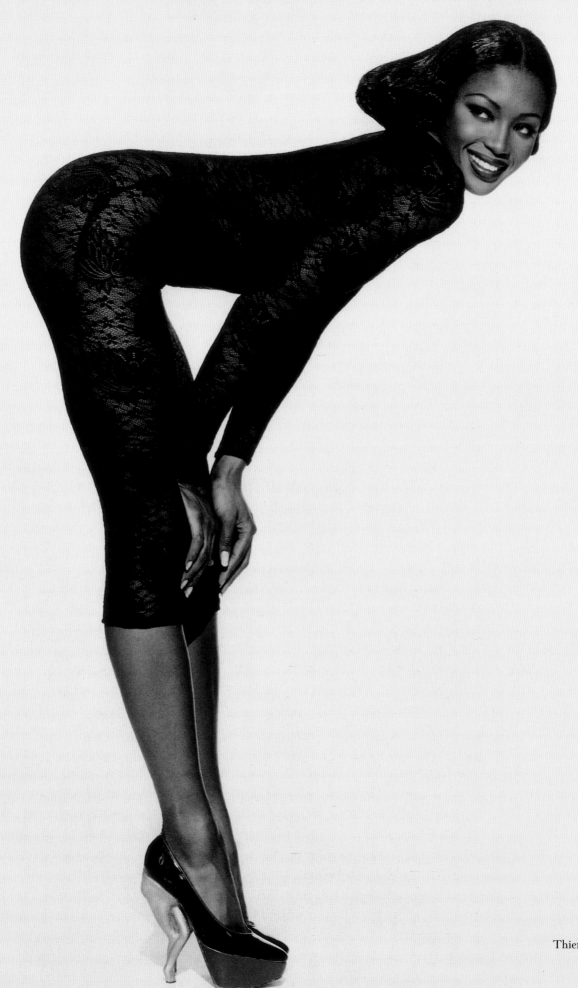

Thierry Le Goüès
1992
Vogue Homme

144

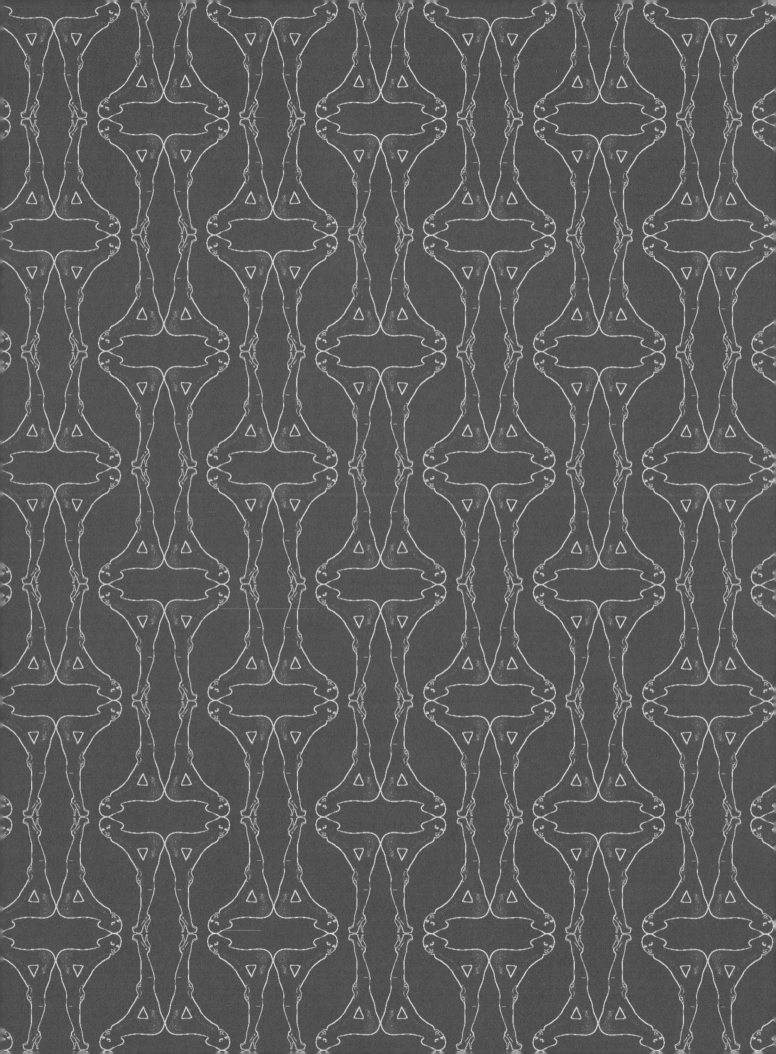